WHAT YOU MUST KNOW ABOUT
BIOIDENTICAL
HORMONE
REPLACEMENT
THERAPY

WHAT YOU MUST KNOW ABOUT
BIOIDENTICAL
HORMONE
REPLACEMENT
THERAPY

AN ALTERNATIVE APPROACH TO EFFECTIVELY TREATING THE SYMPTOMS OF MENOPAUSE

AMY LEE HAWKINS, Pharm.D

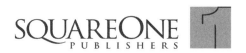

SQUAREONE
PUBLISHERS

COVER DESIGNER: Jeannie Tudor
EDITORS: Michael Weatherhead
TYPESETTER: Gary A. Rosenberg

The information and advice contained in this book are based upon the research and the personal and professional experiences of the author. They are not intended as a substitute for consulting with a health care professional. The publisher and author are not responsible for any adverse effects or consequences resulting from the use of any of the suggestions, preparations, or procedures discussed in this book. All matters pertaining to your physical health should be supervised by a health care professional. It is a sign of wisdom, not cowardice, to seek a second or third opinion.

Square One Publishers
115 Herricks Road
Garden City Park, NY 11040
(516) 535-2010 • (877) 900-BOOK
www.squareonepublishers.com

Library of Congress Cataloging-in-Publication Data
Hawkins, Amy Lee.
  What you must know about bioidentical hormone replacement therapy : an alternative approach to effectively treating the symptoms of menopause / Amy Lee Hawkins.
    p. cm.
  Includes index.
  ISBN 978-0-7570-0380-6
  1. Menopause—Hormone therapy—Popular works. 2. Menopause—Hormone therapy—Complications—Popular works. 3. Middle-aged women—Health and hygiene—Popular works. I. Title. II. Title: Hormone replacement therapy.
  RG186.H395 2013
  618.1'75—dc23
                          2012028419

Printed in the United States of America

10   9   8   7   6   5   4   3   2   1

Contents

3. Bioidentical Hormone Replacement Therapy Guidelines

4. Alternatives to Hormone Replacement Therapy

This book is dedicated to women who are going through perimenopause or menopause, and who may be experiencing hot flashes, night sweats, sleepless nights, mood swings, depression or anxiety, cravings, an expanding waistline, or a diminished sexual appetite.

Here you'll find the answers to your questions regarding bioidentical hormone replacement therapy. You are my inspiration for challenging and educating the medical community on this very controversial topic.

Acknowledgments

I would like thank my family, close friends, and colleagues, without whom this book would not exist. I would particularly like to acknowledge my dad, Ryan, and Mia Jones: Thank you all for your consistent encouragement and support. A special thanks to Karin Craig, the former editor at Sunrise River Press; Kathy Lunniss-Stith, my aunt and high school English teacher; and Heather Reed, a friend and hobbyist screenplay writer; each of whom read my text, corrected my grammar, and provided me with constructive criticism. I would also like to thank Frank Hench, the best pharmacist I know or have had the pleasure of working with, who taught me the art of compounding and introduced me to bioidentical hormone replacement therapy at the inception of my career. Additionally, the American Academy of Anti-Aging Medicine, the Institute for Integrative Medicine, and the Professional Compounding Centers of America are organizations that continually push the envelope in educating the medical community about hormones. By attending many of their conferences, I have been fortunate to meet and learn the latest research from many of the pioneers in bioidentical hormone replacement therapy, including Dr. Jonathan Wright, Dr. James Wilson, and Dr. Pam Smith.

Last but not least, thank you to Square One Publishers for enhancing my manuscript, never accepting less than my best effort, and making this book available to the millions of people who need it.

Preface

I became inspired to write this book while consulting patients on their bioidentical hormone prescriptions. As I explained the basics of bioidentical hormone replacement therapy, all my patients seemed to have very similar questions: What are bioidentical hormones? What are they made of? Will I get cancer if I start taking them? Why do some health professionals discourage their use while others prescribe them? How long will it take for me to feel better? What are the side effects? The conversations became so involved that I began to schedule patients for private sessions to explain to them what hormones are, what each one does, and how to achieve hormonal balance. These consultations took about an hour to discuss the main sex hormones (estrogen, progesterone, and testosterone) and another hour to discuss the metabolic and stress hormones (thyroid, cortisol, DHEA, pregnenolone, melatonin, and human growth hormone). I must have led the same discussion over a hundred times until I realized I could reach more patients in less time if I held community group seminars on BHRT. Soon after this community outreach project started, I was approached by a local CNN news talk radio station to speak on this provocative topic on air each week. It was during this period that I began to write this book.

What You Must Know About Bioidentical Hormone Replacement Therapy is a compilation of all the information I would offer my patients during a consultation. While this book is meant for my patients and other everyday people looking for help, I also wrote it with health professionals in mind. I hope that clinicians might find this book helpful, as it includes recommended hormone dosages, optimal hormone levels, and the key principles required to restore hormonal balance. My overall wish is that people pick up this book, learn from the information it contains, and become experts in bioidentical hormone replacement therapy, extending their knowledge to others who might use it to regain their vitality and a sense of general well-being.

Introduction

For many years, people have been seeking solutions to the various and complex symptoms that accompany the process of aging. Conflicting medical literature (influenced by the money and muscle behind the pharmaceutical industry) has thus far left health care professionals—as well as the people who rely on their advice—baffled, wondering which therapies are sound and which should be avoided. More often than not, physicians prescribe a cocktail of potentially harmful medications that only conceal the symptoms: Prozac for depression, Xanax for anxiety, Ambien for insomnia, Fosamax for osteoporosis, Metformin for high blood sugar, Alli for excess weight, Premarin for hot flashes, and the list goes on. These drugs offer limited relief of pain or discomfort, but they certainly don't address the underlying issues, and they can cause side effects. The fact is that a large number of the health problems associated with getting older are the result of unbalanced or diminished hormone levels. This is particularly true for women, who must inevitably deal with the hormonal fluctuations of menopause.

Prozac helps mask symptoms of irritability and depression, but doesn't address unbalanced hormone levels or the inability to produce enough serotonin, which are the roots of these conditions. Xanax may decrease anxiety, but the real problem may be a

1

lack of progesterone. Similarly, Ambien can help you get some sleep, but recurring night sweats due to low estrogen levels may wake you up. Fosamax increases bone density at first, but may actually increase your risk of fracture over time. Alli may help you lose a couple of pounds, but the underlying cause of your excess weight may be thyroid or adrenal dysfunction. Premarin, an estrogen derived from horses, can alleviate general symptoms of menopause, but this estrogen is a foreign substance to the body, and much more potent than estrogen made naturally by humans. To truly remedy these conditions, it seems obvious that hormonal balance must be restored. But there is so much confusion surrounding hormone replacement therapy that most people don't know what they should do.

In recent years, a form of hormone therapy known as bioidentical hormone replacement therapy has been brought to light as a safe treatment option. Stories on talk shows and in magazines have discussed this treatment only in a superficial way, leaving intelligent people with even more questions that their traditional physicians cannot seem to answer. People still want to know: What exactly are bioidentical hormones? Are they all hype, or can they actually help? Are they the same as natural hormones? Are they safe? Who's a candidate for treatment? What is the standard duration of therapy? What are the common side effects of these products? Will they help with weight control, mood, and energy level? The purpose of this book is to answer these and a myriad of other related questions.

If you are a woman entering menopause, this book will allow you to navigate this phase of life more comfortably and healthfully. It provides a detailed explanation of the menstrual cycle, all the hormones it affects, and how this process changes over the years. You'll also become acquainted with the hormones behind stress, metabolism, energy, and mood. Before long, you will have a rich understanding of your body's delicate hormonal balance and its intricate hormonal fluctuations. At this point, you will learn how to achieve optimal hormone levels through bioidentical hormone replacement therapy. But whether or not you choose hormone replacement therapy, this book also outlines many other treatment options, including vitamins and other supplements, and dietary and lifestyle changes that can benefit your well-being enormously.

If you've been desperately searching for a way to alleviate symptoms of hormonal imbalance without a handful of drugs or a regimen of hormone replacements that aren't quite the same as what your body used to make naturally, *What You Must Know About Bioidentical Hormone Replacement Therapy* is the guide book for you. Reading this book and talking about bioidentical hormone replacement therapy with a progressive health practitioner can help you learn the advantages and risks involved with this type of treatment, allowing you to decide if it is the right choice for your body.

1

Introducing Your Hormones

Hormones are chemical substances that act as messengers between cells. They carry signals that tell cells what to do. Essentially, without instructions from hormones, cells would become confused and begin to malfunction. Hormones are made mainly in endocrine glands and control important cellular processes, including hair growth, bone formation, and biological transitions such as puberty and menopause. Each type of hormone is matched to a unique hormone receptor located on the surface of a cell, and fits into its receptor like a key into a lock. Once a hormone "unlocks" a cell, it is able to transmit its message. A hormone may, for example, tell a cell to replicate, make a certain protein, or increase energy production.

When hormones leave glands and travel to their target cells or tissues, some of them hitch a ride with a protein, while others make the trip on their own. If a hormone is carried by a protein, it is not free to communicate with a cell until it is released. A hormone that circulates freely through the blood, however, can affect a cell immediately.

But how does the body know when to make hormones? First, the brain senses that the body is low on a particular hormone. It then sends a message to the gland that makes this hormone, which subsequently produces this substance in the required amount. Finally, a part of the brain called the hypothalamus detects when enough hormone has been created and signals the gland to stop production until levels fall again.

Although they affect hundreds of biological functions, the hormones estrogen, testosterone, and progesterone are primarily considered sex hormones because they control sexual development and fertility. In addition, other major hormones, including melatonin, DHEA, insulin, and cortisol, influence physiological processes such as mood regulation, metabolism, energy production, and the ability to cope with stress. Learning the roles that hormones play in the body is an important step toward recognizing when they are not working right. Moreover, understanding how certain hormones affect each other can provide another important piece of the biological puzzle. Once you have the right information, you may be able to identify which hormones are out of balance and take steps to remedy the problem.

■ CORTISOL

Produced in the adrenal glands, cortisol is a steroid hormone predominantly known for its relationship to stress. It is released in reaction to danger and initiates the body's fight-or-flight response. In other words, cortisol prepares the body to fight off a predator or run away from it. If, for example, you were to come face to face with a bear, no doubt your cortisol level would soar. It would then stimulate an increase in blood sugar (released from muscle) and fatty acid levels, blood flow to muscle, strength, blood pressure, heart rate and contractility, pupil dilation, the opening of the airways, mental activity, and your metabolic rate. All this happens so that you can either fight the bear or run away quickly. Additionally, cortisol is meant for other acutely stressful situations like dehydration, injury, infection, low blood sugar, or the ingestion of toxins. Although this hormone helps to block the sensation of pain during stressful situations, it also takes the body's focus away from processes like reproduction, digestion, growth, energy storage, and sleep.

Aside from its role in stress reactions, cortisol influences mood, thoughts, weight, bone density, the immune system, protein production, hormonal balance, and fetal development. It is such an important hormone, in fact, that life cannot continue even one day without it. Cortisol levels are normally at their highest in the morning, helping the body wake up and prepare for the day. They then steadily decline into the evening. By bedtime, the amount of cortisol in the blood is typically low. Interestingly, while the production of other hormones tends to decrease over time, cortisol levels actually tend to increase with age, particularly if you lead a stressful life.

While cortisol was meant to provide the body with an appropriate way to deal with the acutely stressful situations of the distant past, such as being attacked by an animal, how often do you come face to face with a predator and need to run or fight for your life these days? The truth is that modern stress comes from family issues, work, finances, chronic disease, and other pressures. The problem is that cortisol does not differentiate stressors. Whether the stressor is a real emergency, such as a car accident, or a perceived one, such as worrying about what someone thinks of you, the body's response is the same. Because modern stress affects the body daily, the stress reaction can become chronic. Unfortunately, the body does a poor job of managing chronic stress. Over time, chronic stress can have a negative affect on adrenal gland function and lead to hormonal imbalance.

Chronically Elevated Cortisol

Today, the fast pace and heavy demands of work life, family life, and social life put excessive stress on many individuals every day. Instead of producing cortisol to handle a quick burst of stress and then going back to normal, the body makes more and more of this hormone to deal with these constant worries and pressures. As such, cortisol levels remain elevated throughout the day. Meanwhile, other hormone production is put on the back burner, which creates further hormonal imbalances.

Many harmful effects are associated with chronically elevated cortisol. Remember, cortisol's job includes ensuring that energy stores are ready to use on demand in the face of danger. This increases glucose and fats in the blood stream, which, if allowed to stay elevated, can lead to diabetes or insulin resistance as well as high cholesterol. Unfortunately, glucose is best absorbed by fat cells in the belly, which means that chronically raised cortisol can also cause an increased waistline. Cortisol often steals protein from muscle in order to make more glucose, too, resulting in loss of muscle tissue.

In addition to its effect on glucose levels, cortisol also affects the cardiovascular system. It causes blood vessels in the muscles to dilate, blood pressure and heart rate to increase, and makes the heart contract more strongly so that the body can get ready to run or fight. Chronically elevated cortisol, therefore, can lead to high blood pressure and heart disease.

Since the body is not concerned with blood flow to the genitals or hormonal balance in times of increased cortisol production, impotence and reproductive issues can be a problem in women and men with chronically raised levels of this hormone. It also causes blood to leave the gut and kidneys and move towards the muscles, which leads to impaired digestion, irritable bowel, water retention, and electrolyte disturbances. In a real emergency, water retention is a good idea because blood volume increases, adding protection if you became badly wounded. But when this reaction occurs on a regular basis, it encourages hypertension and disturbs the balance of electrolytes in the body, as potassium, magnesium, and calcium levels drop. This calcium deficit increases the risk of osteoporosis, as the body does not build bone during times of cortisol production and may actually leach calcium from bone to make up for the recent decrease in this mineral. And since cortisol discourages growth, human growth hormone production decreases, resulting in further loss of muscle tissue. Furthermore, the elevated blood flow to muscle creates unused lactic acid, which can build up and cause achy muscles in a condition commonly known as fibromyalgia.

But these are not the only results of chronically elevated cortisol. Other metabolic problems also occur. For example, the hormones norepinephrine and epinephrine become responsible for energy and metabolism, while thyroid hormones take a back seat in the process. One consequence of this change is weight gain. In addition, when demand for norepinephrine and epinephrine goes up, production of the neurotransmitters serotonin and dopamine goes down, leading to anxiety and depression over time. Lastly, because the immune system is not needed in a real emergency, cortisol shuts it down. Thus, infections become more capable of leading to illness during chronic periods of stress.

Symptoms of High Cortisol

The following symptoms are typical of someone with high cortisol levels. If you have more than half of these symptoms, it is likely that your cortisol production is elevated to an unhealthy degree:

- Diabetes and insulin resistance

- Difficulty losing weight

- Excess facial and body hair

- Excessive bruising

- Fatigue

- Feeling anxious or depressed

- Fibromyalgia (achy joints and muscles)

- Heart disease and increased cholesterol

- Impotence and decreased sex drive

- Infections and decreased immunity

- Infertility and infrequent periods

- Inflammatory bowel and digestive problems

- Lowered ability to activate thyroid hormones

- Memory loss

- Osteoporosis

- Problems sleeping or sleep apnea
- Severe PMS and menopause symptoms
- Sodium and water retention
- Thin skin and stretch marks
- Weight gain, especially around your waist

According to the American Institute of Stress, "Stress is the underlying cause of 75 to 90 percent of all primary care visits." The statement is bold, yet the list of most commonly prescribed drugs shows how true it is. High blood pressure, high cholesterol, heart disease, diabetes, stomach upset, hormonal issues, pain, and depression are among today's most commonly diagnosed disease states. These conditions can directly arise from dealing with chronic stress. Unfortunately, writing a quick prescription to address chronic disease states like these addresses only the symptoms and not the underlying cause. Ultimately, if cortisol is allowed to remain elevated, it can lead to an entirely new stage of illness called adrenal fatigue.

Adrenal Fatigue

If chronic stress and elevated cortisol levels are allowed to continue for years, the adrenal glands will grow tired from making excessive amounts of this hormone. It is then that you will experience what is called adrenal fatigue, which is when the adrenal glands shut down and cortisol levels plummet. This condition can harm your immune system and actually be life-threatening. Without cortisol, the immune system is forced to work overtime, which can lead to autoimmune diseases like rheumatoid arthritis or lupus. At this point, cortisol therapy may be essential.

Dr. Hans Seyle, a noted Canadian endocrinologist, has described the way in which most people reach adrenal fatigue as a progression through the following three stages.

Alarm Reaction

A severely stressful period, such as a divorce, death in the family, or sudden increase in work demands, results in the fight-or-flight response. Cortisol levels rise to provide you extra energy to cope with the situation. If the stress continues, however, the brain and adrenal glands will find a way to make more and more cortisol, eventually stealing from other hormone stores (especially DHEA and pregnenolone).

Resistance Stage

A stressful life means your brain and adrenals must work overtime to maintain a high cortisol output and remain on constant alert. Gradually, though, the adrenals stop listening to the brain's signals and begin to produce less cortisol—they can't keep up with the constant demand. This is the resistance stage. If the stress passes, you can start to rebuild your defenses and store energy.

A Glimpse of Adrenal Fatigue

The day starts at 7:30 AM as you hit the snooze button several times before you can muster enough energy to roll out of the bed. You get up and go through your morning routine, but feel very tired despite the reasonable amount of sleep you just had. Maybe you just aren't a morning person? So you head down to the coffee shop for your latte and scone and then to the office. While at work, you finally feel like you are awake around 10:00 AM. Your boss hands you a new account to work on, but you could care less. It just takes so much effort to go above and beyond like you used to. Work goes on, lunch with your coworkers passes (you only feel like eating a few chips because you have indigestion), and then 3:00 PM hits. You feel like you felt this morning, so you reach for a chocolate bar or maybe an energy drink to get through the workday. After dinner, though, you are feeling surprisingly good. You watch a few shows to get into sleep mode. It's 10:00 PM now and you're tired, but something tells you it's not time yet. So you flip through that murder mystery novel you've been hooked on and before you know it, it's 1:00 AM! Oh well, maybe tomorrow you'll get it right.

If the stress is prolonged, you will transition to the next stage. How long it takes to become exhausted depends on your genes, diet, exercise, sleep patterns, and stress-management skills.

Exhaustion Stage

After years of stress, your cortisol storage is now depleted and your adrenals have quit on you. You are officially burned out and have succumbed to adrenal fatigue. Cortisol levels are typically low throughout both day and night. The negative results are widespread. You have no energy, simple tasks are difficult to complete, all major hormones are either low or unbalanced, and many chronic disease states may have developed along the way.

If you have more than half of the following symptoms, it is likely that you have already gone through the first two stages and are now suffering from adrenal fatigue:

- Chronic fatigue and muscle weakness

- Constipation or diarrhea under stress

- Cravings for salty and high-fat foods

- Decreased ability to handle stress

- Decreased sex drive

- Depression

- Increased allergies

- Increased effort to do everyday tasks

- Increased incidence of diabetes, fibromyalgia, or anorexia

- Increased PMS or menopausal symptoms

- Intolerance to high-potassium foods in the morning (fruit)

- Lightheadedness when rising

- Liver spots

- Low blood sugar

- Lowered resistance to infections

- Respiratory conditions

- Swollen ankles in the morning

- Use of caffeine or sugar to drive yourself

The fact is that the best prescription for stress relief is not a pill, but rather lifestyle changes and coping skills. There are, however, some supplements that can also help the adrenal glands regain proper function and balance. (See pages 109 and 161.)

■ DEHYDROEPIANDROSTERONE (DHEA)

Dehydroepiandrosterone (DHEA) is the most abundant hormone in the body. Considered the "Fountain of Youth," this steroid hormone synthesizes testosterone, estrogen, and progesterone, and has cardiovascular, metabolic, and anti-stress qualities. It is made in the adrenal glands, skin, and brain, and actually helps reverse the effects of stress on the immune system while decreasing excess cortisol levels. When DHEA levels are optimal, its benefits can be seen throughout the body in the following ways:

- **Cardiovascular.** Decreases cholesterol, prevents clotting of the blood, and lowers triglycerides.

- **Metabolic.** Decreases the storage of fat, promotes weight loss and lean muscle mass, increases basal metabolic rate, and encourages insulin sensitivity.

- **Neurological.** Increases brain function (including memory), helps regulate mood and alleviate depression, increases serotonin (a neurotransmitter that improves mood, prevents anxiety, and stops food cravings), lowers the perception of stress (it decreases and antagonizes cortisol), improves sleep, and protects neurons from injury and degradation.

In addition to these effects, DHEA raises human growth hormone levels, enhances longevity, increases bone formation and density, promotes fertility, helps maintain pregnancy, reverses vaginal thinning, improves libido, supports immunity, discourages cancer cell replication, helps treat fibromyalgia, increases skin thickness, prevents dry skin, decreases skin pigmentation, stimulates collagen synthesis, and promotes wound healing.

Interestingly, no DHEA receptors have yet been found in the body. Researchers currently believe that DHEA functions primarily as a reservoir for the production of sex hormones. Unlike with other hormones, there is no biological system that senses the supply and demand of DHEA. Thus, if you are deficient in DHEA because of stress or aging, you will remain so until you take supplemental DHEA or minimize your stress level. Because this substance converts into sex hormones, however, it is important that you do not use supplemental DHEA when it is not truly needed. It can increase testosterone in women and estrogen in men, which may lead to further hormonal imbalances. Therefore, it is important to recognize the symptoms of both low DHEA and excess DHEA.

Symptoms of Low DHEA

It is not clear if DHEA supplementation can improve the diseases associated with low DHEA levels. Hormone testing is a great way to confirm whether your levels are optimal. (See page 80.) If you have more than half of the symptoms or conditions on this list, you probably don't make enough DHEA:

- Autoimmune disease, such as lupus or rheumatoid arthritis
- Breast and ovarian cancers
- Chronic fatigue syndrome
- Depression
- Diabetes (type II)
- Dry skin
- Heart disease
- High blood pressure
- Immune deficiencies
- Lack of libido
- Osteoporosis
- Weight gain, trouble losing weight, or obesity

The primary two causes of low DHEA are aging and chronic stress. In the elderly, it is common to see DHEA levels decline by up to 74 percent. But low levels of DHEA can also result from smoking over a long period of time. This is because nicotine can prevent the formation of the enzyme needed to make DHEA. You can't change your age, but you can quit smoking, improve your response to stress, exercise more, and consume less calories to jumpstart your natural DHEA production. If these methods are not sufficient, DHEA replacement therapy can be put to use. (See page 101.)

Symptoms of High DHEA

If you have more than half of the symptoms on this list, it is likely your DHEA level is too high:

- Abnormal periods
- Acne
- Hair on chin and upper lip of females
- Headache
- Heart palpitations
- Increased perspiration
- Insomnia
- Male pattern baldness
- Nasal congestion
- Oily hair
- Oily skin
- Skin rash

If your DHEA level is found to be naturally high, there are a few things you can do to help lower it. First, measure your levels of estrogen and progesterone. They may be found to be too low, and supplementing them to restore balance may also help decrease excess DHEA. Additionally, cutting down on animal protein in your diet and adding a vitamin E supplement to your daily regimen can help balance DHEA. Lastly, if you take supplemental DHEA and find that your levels are high, you obviously need to decrease your dosage.

■ ESTROGEN

Estrogen has more than 400 functions and affects every cell of the body, including skin, hair, bone, heart, and brain cells. Classified as a steroid hormone, estrogen is mainly known for causing the body to develop female characteristics during puberty. It also balances the actions of the hormone progesterone. A woman's body makes three types of estrogen: estrone (E1), estradiol (E2), and estriol (E3). These estrogens are produced directly by the ovaries and indirectly by other tissues such as body fat. While a man's body also synthesizes a certain amount of estradiol, estrogen is understandably found in much larger amounts in women.

Recognizing the symptoms of estrogen imbalance will certainly come in handy to a woman as she progresses through the different stages of her life, and understanding the three kinds of natural estrogen can provide even more help.

Estrone (E1)

While estrone has benefits like reducing risk of osteoporosis, its association with breast cancer is strong. It is found in fatty tissue and is still made even after menopause, typically from androgens like testosterone. Women who are overweight and have a high percentage of body fat tend to experience fewer symptoms of menopause because their estrone levels are high enough. Some overweight women, however, find their body fat provides insulation that leads to a higher body temperature and thus more hot flashes.

Estradiol (E2)

The strongest estrogen, estradiol, gives you feminine features and promotes youthful skin, thick hair, and beautiful curves. It also builds bone, encourages insulin sensitivity, decreases LDL cholesterol (also known as bad cholesterol), and has many more benefits. Its drawback is an association with breast cancer if present in elevated levels.

Estriol (E3)

Estriol functions similarly to estradiol, but it is weaker and may be protective against breast cancer. It is commonly paired with estradiol hormone replacement to protect against breast cancer growth. For those with an excess of estrogen, supplementing with estriol is like taking an anti-estrogen medication. Estriol occupies the estrogen receptor, taking the place of more potent estrogens. Some European clinics have used estriol as part of a breast cancer treatment protocol instead of tamoxifen, a chemotherapy agent. Another popular application of estriol is to apply it to the vaginal wall, where estriol receptors are abundant, which can greatly alleviate vaginal dryness. One drawback is that estriol supplementation may add a couple of pounds to your hips and thighs if you take too much.

Estrogen Balance

An optimal estrogen level, balanced correctly with other hormones, benefits the body in many ways, including the following:

- **Cardiovascular.** Decreases LDL cholesterol and increases HDL cholesterol (also known as good cholesterol), lessens the risk of heart disease, decreases arterial plaque buildup, reduces inflammatory effects of cholesterol, lowers blood pressure, opens small arteries, preserves artery elasticity, enhances blood flow, and prevents blood clotting.

- **Dental.** Helps prevent tooth loss.

- **Dermatological.** Retains collagen in the skin, boosts the water content of the skin, helps maintain tone and softness, and decreases the appearance of wrinkles.

- **Metabolic.** Improves metabolism, increases energy, promotes insulin sensitivity, and regulates body temperature.

- **Musculoskeletal.** Sustains muscle tissue, guards against muscle damage, and prevents bone loss.

- **Neurological.** Indirectly reduces risk of Alzheimer's disease, improves sleep, improves memory, enhances reasoning and concentration, improves mood, heightens fine motor skills, produces nerve growth factor, aids in the formation of serotonin.

- **Ocular.** Reduces the risk of cataracts and guards against glaucoma and macular degeneration.

- **Miscellaneous.** Decreases the risk of colon cancer, acts as an antioxidant, reduces homocysteine (an amino acid derivative that promotes cardiovascular disease), and increases sexual interest.

Estrogen levels can be too low, particularly as a woman approaches menopause, leading to a variety of symptoms and health problems. If you experience signs and symptoms of low estrogen and have laboratory test results confirming abnormal levels, you may be a candidate for bioidentical estrogen replacement therapy. (See page 88.)

Symptoms of Low Estrogen

The following are the typical symptoms a woman experiences when her estrogen level is low. If you have more than half of these conditions, you probably have an estrogen imbalance:

- Bone loss
- Decreased skin tone
- Dry skin and eyes
- Headaches
- Heart palpitations
- Hot flashes
- Insomnia or daytime sleepiness
- Leaky bladder (urinary incontinence)
- Light, sporadic, or no periods
- Low sex drive
- Memory loss or "brain fog"
- Mood disturbances (depression or anxiety)
- Night sweats
- Osteoporosis
- Pain during intercourse
- Thinning hair

- Vaginal dryness

- Worsening asthma

- Wrinkles (fine vertical lines above lips)

- Yeast infections

If you suspect that you might have a problem with your estrogen level, hormone testing is a great way to confirm if your levels are not optimal. (See page 80).

Symptoms of High Estrogen

Throughout life, estrogen levels can also become too high relative to other hormones. This hormonal imbalance is called estrogen dominance. Estrogen dominance is found particularly in women during adolescence and at the onset of menopause, which is called perimenopause.

The following are the typical symptoms a woman experiences when her estrogen levels are high. The more of these conditions you have, the more likely it is that your estrogen is out of balance:

- Achy joints

- Bloating

- Breast tenderness

- Cold body temperature

- Craving sweets or carbohydrates

- Excessive or irregular bleeding or spotting between periods

- Fatigue

- Fibrocyctic breasts

- Hair loss on the scalp

- Headaches

- Irritable moods

- Uterine fibroids

- Weight gain

It is important to note that American women tend to experience this imbalance more often than women of other countries. This is likely because American women generally eat a diet low in fiber and high in fat (yet low in omega-3 fatty acids), and don't exercise regularly. It may also be due to an elevated exposure to estrogen-mimicking substances called xenoestrogens, which can wreak havoc on your health.

What Are Xenoestrogens?

All blood passes through the liver, which removes toxins that have entered the body through food or exposure to chemicals. Estrogens, whether from the body's glands or from supplements, enter the bloodstream and pass through the liver, where they are chopped into smaller bits called metabolites. This process makes them water soluble so excess hormones can be excreted through the urine.

Some of these metabolites are useful, but others can promote cancer at high levels. For example, estrone can be broken down into the metabolites 6-alpha-OH estrone and 4-OH estrone. The metabolites are examples of xenoestrogens, which are substances that look similar to natural estrogens. Like a wolf in sheep's clothing, they can still bind to a cell's estrogen receptors, but confuse cells by giving them different messages. Over time, they can lead to cancer by telling cells to multiply too often. They may also promote allergies and infections, and affect reproduction, metabolism, and stress tolerance. Whether the breakdown of estrogen produces useful or harmful metabolites depends on a person's genes, exposure level to toxins, and liver health.

Not all xenoestrogens, however, come from the body's metabolism of estrogen. Others are created by lifestyle and daily exposure to certain outside substances.

Sources of Xenoestrogens

It is important to recognize all sources of xenoestrogens and avoid them whenever possible. If you are regularly exposed to the following substances, your body may already be dealing with the effects of xenoestrogens:

- Birth control pills
- Caffeine

- Cosmetics that contain DMDM hydantoin, imidazolidinyl urea, fragrance, dyes, methylchloroisothiazolinone, methylisothiazolinone, parabens, PEG, sodium lauryl or laureth sulfate, triclosan, triclocarban, or triethanolamine

- Chronic consumption of alcohol

- Conjugated equine estrogens

- Food microwaved in plastic containers

- Industrial air pollution

- Pesticides

- Plastics

- Processed or high-fat foods

- Synthetic hormones and antibiotics fed to farm animals

- Tap water

Other factors such as lack of exercise, obesity, smoking, and stress also promote xenoestrogenic activity in the body, leading to an overload of these toxic substances. When the liver becomes overwhelmed with xenoestrogens, its ability to dispose of these hormone-mimickers is negatively affected, which can result in a toxic buildup.

Xenoestrogen Detoxification

If an accumulation of xenoestrogens is suspected, it may be helpful to measure levels with a twenty-four-hour urine collection test. If the results are positive, you may be able to lower the amount of these toxins in your system by taking an extract called diindolylmethane (DIM). DIM is the active metabolite of indole-3-carbinol, which facilitates elimination of xenoestrogens and is found in foods such as broccoli, cabbage, Brussels sprouts, cauliflower, and kale. Prescription DIM is recommended instead of over-the-counter supplements that contain DIM, which have a much lower dose of the substance and usually do not have verified purity. A month of DIM at 150 to 300 mg daily should produce benefits, but ongoing supplementation may be better. A follow-up urinalysis will help determine how to proceed. At the therapeutic dosage, DIM can cause headaches and sometimes a rash for the first few weeks of use, but these go away as the estrogenic toxins are cleared out.

It is worth noting that I do recommend the use of DIM to men as well as women. As they age, men can develop high estrogen levels, often due to xenoestrogens. Taking DIM can lower the amount of these toxins in a man's body and possibly even relieve associated prostate issues.

Milk thistle is a liver detoxification herb that goes hand in hand with DIM supplementation. If you have used this therapy to rid your body of xenoestrogens, it is very important that you undergo a three-week course of milk thistle to clean out your liver. I recommend 220 mg of milk thistle three times daily for three to four weeks. You can find this product over the counter at most pharmacies.

Besides DIM and milk thistle, there are other supplements that can help protect you from xenoestrogen buildup, including soy isoflavones, flaxseed, omega-3 fatty acids, methionine, magnesium, vitamin B_2 (riboflavin), vitamin B_6 (pyridoxine), vitamin B_{12} (methylcobalamin), folic acid or folinic acid (the more active form of folic acid), glycine, glutamate, rosemary, turmeric, and antioxidants such as vitamin C, vitamin E, glutathione, and melatonin. Your doctor can help decide which supplements would be best for your situation.

Another way to detoxify the liver is through the use of substances known as methyl donors. Methyl donors attach to other compounds, making them more water soluble and therefore easier to eliminate through the urine. Methyl donors include S-adenosyl-L-methionine (SAMe), methylsulfonylmethane (MSM), betaine, and methyltetrahydrofolate (MTHF). If you are lacking in these substances, you are most likely not metabolizing estrogen properly, causing it to build up in your tissues. Fortunately, you can take the previously mentioned methyl donors as over-the-counter supplements to aid in estrogen metabolism.

While supplements can help your liver detoxify, you still need to take control of your diet and lifestyle to minimize xenoestrogen exposure. Try to avoid anything that contributes to the problem. Eat whole foods (preferably organic) that are rich in protein and omega-3 fatty acids (for example, flaxseed and fish oil) and free from chemicals, minimize intake of omega-6 fatty acids (found in most fried foods), exercise regularly, don't microwave food in plastic containers, limit caffeine and alcohol consumption, stop smoking, and drink clean, filtered water. You may well experience other benefits by adopting these changes, like a shrinking waistline or a more restful night's sleep!

■ HUMAN GROWTH HORMONE (hGH)

The pituitary gland secretes human growth hormone (hGH) about five times a day. The main functions of hGH are to stimulate growth and development in maturing children. In addition, it supports the immune system, cellular rejuvenation, tissue repair, wound healing, bone density and strength, brain function, and skin, hair, and nail strength. Finally, this hormone also plays a metabolic role, increasing muscle mass, promoting the breakdown of fat, and generating glucose for energy.

As with other hormones, human growth hormone levels peak during the teens, and then drop each subsequent year. In fact, beyond the age of twenty-one, hGH naturally decreases 50 percent every seven years. Exposure to certain substances such as xenoestrogens and other chemicals found in plastics can also cause hGH levels to fall. This drop in human growth hormone leads to a higher percentage of body fat and decreased bone density.

Symptoms of Low hGH

If you have more than half of the symptoms listed, you probably have adult growth hormone deficiency. Curiously, symptoms of growth hormone deficiency are often similar to those of excess cortisol, and include the following:

- Cardiovascular disease
- Decreased cognition
- Emotional problems
- High serum lipid concentrations
- Increased fat mass (especially around waist)
- Lack of energy and vitality
- Loss of muscle and strength
- Low bone density
- Lowered confidence
- Lowered immune function
- Poor exercise capacity
- Reduced vigor and optimism
- Sexual dysfunction

The effects of low hGH, which are generally considered unavoidable aspects of growing older, have led researchers to wonder whether supplementation might be an appropriate treatment for aging. (See page 102.) Research conducted by Dr. Daniel Rudman in 1990 reported human growth hormone's positive effects on a small group of older men. This and many other studies support the idea that hGH supplementation leads to an increase in lean body mass and bone density, and a decrease in fat mass. More recently, human growth hormone has been used experimentally to treat multiple sclerosis, AIDS, fibromyalgia, heart failure, and certain gastrointestinal disorders. On the flip side, it has also been abused by athletes to enhance their performance.

■ INSULIN

Produced by the pancreas, insulin is a hormone that regulates blood sugar levels in the body. It enables cells to convert glucose, also known as sugar, into energy. Without insulin, the body would not be able to harness dietary glucose for energy, thus allowing it to build up in the blood. When blood glucose levels are too high, the pancreas must secrete more insulin to balance them. Over time, this leads to a metabolic condition called insulin resistance (also called metabolic syndrome or metabolic syndrome X), in which cells are no longer able to use insulin properly.

To better understand how this condition occurs, imagine that you live in a muscle cell and that insulin is a delivery person who brings you your necessary glucose at every meal. When the delivery person shows up, you open the muscle cell door, take the glucose inside, and become full and energized. Lately, however, the delivery person has been receiving large, more frequent shipments of glucose from the gut. There are now more meals to deliver to the cells, and additional delivery workers are needed to keep up with all the shipments.

The delivery person begins to show up at your door with glucose twice as often. You take the extra meals inside, but you're not really hungry. Boxes of glucose begin to pile up in the kitchen. Every time a delivery appears, you try not to let the glucose in, but it keeps coming. Gradually, the muscle cell overflows with stocks of glucose. So, one day, you turn out all the lights, and when insulin knocks on the door, you pretend you're not home, preventing glucose from entering. In other words, you have developed insulin resistance.

The delivery person doesn't know what to do with all the glucose. Luckily, there is a party going on at the fat cell just down the street. Loads of people are there and they are happy to take all the glucose insulin has to offer so they can convert it into fat. The party's host tells the delivery person to bring glucose there anytime because everyone there is always hungry. Insulin still visits muscle cells, but since there are so many glucose shipments, it starts a new relationship with fat cells, so that all the surplus glucose can be dropped off at these locations.

If this cycle is allowed to persist, the body will not be able to metabolize glucose at all. This condition is called diabetes. Thankfully, there are ways to reverse insulin resistance and avoid full-blown diabetes before it sets in. (See page 133.)

■ MELATONIN

Melatonin is a sleep-promoting hormone secreted by the pineal gland in the brain. It is also a powerful antioxidant that improves mood, immunity, and tolerance to stress; combats premature aging, stimulates human growth hormone production, decreases cortisol levels, and regulates other hormones.

Nighttime darkness spurs production of melatonin, while daylight suppresses its activity. As such, those who are blind, work nights, or have jet lag may have disrupted melatonin cycles. While young children have the highest amounts of nighttime melatonin, these levels diminish with advancing age. Many elderly people experience interrupted sleep and tend to wake up earlier than when they were younger simply because their melatonin level is too low.

In addition to insomnia, low melatonin levels have been associated with health conditions such as depression and breast cancer. Taking melatonin supplements, however, may help alleviate or avoid these issues. (See page 109.)

■ PREGNENOLONE

Synthesized from cholesterol, pregnenolone is a prohormone, or precursor hormone, of many steroid hormones. It is the starting point for the creation of progesterone, DHEA, estrogen, testosterone, and cortisol. It is produced not only in the adrenals and ovaries, but also in the brain and spinal cord. It enhances memory and cognition, counteracts fatigue and stress, alleviates arthritis pain, repairs nerve damage, reduces the risk of dementia, promotes brain cell formation, helps you sleep, lowers cholesterol, supports vision and hearing, is a natural antidepressant, and can increase longevity. At low doses it can relax you; at high doses it can energize you.

Since levels of pregnenolone decline with age, many anti-aging clinicians use pregnenolone supplementation to slow the aging process. Since pregnenolone is a prohormone, some believe that the body converts it into whichever hormone is lacking in order to restore hormonal balance. For example, they believe that if you give pregnenolone to a woman who is low in estrogen, her body will convert pregnenolone into the required amount of estrogen. Other physicians, however, believe that only the specific hormones that are lacking should be used to address a hormonal imbalance. I agree with this second approach, mainly because genes influence which hormone is made by pregnenolone. They could, therefore, synthesize this prohormone into something the body does not need. For example, if you are low in progesterone and take pregnenolone to increase progesterone levels, your body may have other plans and convert pregnenolone to estrogen instead. So, if you are low in progesterone, supplement with progesterone. Supplement with pregnenolone only when this particular hormone is low.

Pregnenolone should remain at its optimal level in the blood, which is between 100 and 170 ng/dL (nanograms per deciliter) for both women and men. If your level falls within this ideal range, there should not be a need to supplement. Aging, stress, and adrenal fatigue, however, can lower pregnenolone under the recommended amount, causing symptoms such as impaired memory, moodiness, and decreased energy. At this point, supplements can be taken. Otherwise, estrogen deficiency or low testosterone levels may follow. Be cautious before self-treating low pregnenolone levels, however, as over-the-counter preparations vary widely in dosage, from 5 to 150 mg or more. If you wish to try over-the-counter pregnenolone, choose one from a high-quality company with proven potency standardization methods and start with a low dose. (See page 110.) As always, it is best to meet with an experienced health care practitioner to decide the proper regimen for your situation.

■ PROGESTERONE

Although progesterone balances the actions of estrogen and affects the health of your skin, hair, bones, heart, and brain, its main purpose is to maintain pregnancy and ensure that a fetus is carried to term. Women synthesize progesterone in the ovaries and adrenal glands. During pregnancy, it is also produced in the placenta. Men produce this hormone in the testicles and adrenal glands, only in much smaller amounts than women.

Progesterone is an amazing hormone that, like estrogen, acts on every single cell in the body. When progesterone is in balance with the body's other hormones, it can produce many kinds of benefits, including the following:

- **Anti-Cancer.** Reduces the risk of breast cancer.

- **Cardiovascular.** Lowers blood pressure and cholesterol, normalizes blood clotting, and reduces inflammation.

- **Dermatological.** Increases hair on the scalp and maintains elasticity of the skin.

- **Metabolic.** Burns fat for energy, increases metabolism, promotes insulin secretion in response to glucose, acts as a natural diuretic, and helps eliminate bloating.

- **Musculoskeletal.** Builds bone (while estrogen only prevents bone loss) and helps relieve the symptoms of arthritis.

- **Neurological.** Decreases anxiety and depression, improves sleep, helps manage mood, may decrease the number of epileptic seizures, may alleviate headaches, promotes the myelination of neurons (protects brain tissue).

Progesterone also balances the effects of estrogen, helps promote estrogen metabolism (which prevents estrogen dominance and protects the uterus), improves libido, prevents hot flashes, and promotes longevity. Unfortunately, many women don't have enough of this hormone, and clinicians may fail to detect the deficiency.

Symptoms of Low Progesterone

Progesterone is the hormone that drops first during perimenopause, causing many of the related symptoms. Progesterone levels may become too low during this stage of life and beyond, but the problem can occur in young ladies as well. Besides perimenopause, there are other causes of low progesterone, such as breastfeeding, chronic stress, antidepressant use, arginine consumption (seen in body builders and weight-loss clinics), a diet high in refined sugars and saturated fat, impaired thyroid function, and vitamin A, B, and C deficiencies.

The following are the typical symptoms a woman experiences when her progesterone levels are low, a few of which are also common symptoms of premenstrual syndrome. These conditions include the following:

- Adrenal fatigue
- Anxiety
- Arthritis
- Bloating
- Bleeding between periods
- Cramps
- Decreased HDL
- Decreased sex drive
- Endometriosis (when uterine cells start to grow outside the uterus)
- Estrogen dominance symptoms
- Hard to reach climax
- Heavy, frequent, or irregular periods
- Hot flashes
- Inflammation and pain
- Insomnia
- Irritability or mood swings
- Leaking urine
- Osteoporosis
- Polycystic ovarian syndrome (PCOS, a disorder associated with obesity, excess masculine hormones, and irregular periods)
- Weight gain
- Wrinkled or drooping skin

If you experience symptoms of low progesterone, and the levels are confirmed, you may be a candidate for progesterone replacement therapy. (See page 90.)

Symptoms of High Progesterone

If you've been pregnant, then you've surely experienced symptoms of progesterone excess. A placenta makes as much as 400 mg of progesterone each day, which is ten to fifteen times the normal amount made by the ovaries. The following are the typical symptoms a woman experiences when her progesterone levels are high:

- Achy joints
- Acne
- Breast swelling
- Decreased glucose tolerance
- Depression
- Difficulty losing weight
- Excessive sleep or daytime sleepiness
- Facial hair
- Fatigue
- Increased appetite (and carbohydrate cravings)
- Increased insulin resistance
- Nausea
- Nipple tenderness or itching
- Yeast overgrowth

Usually pregnancy is the only time a woman would experience signs of progesterone excess, but check the list of symptoms if you are taking progesterone replacement therapy. If a number of them apply to you, you may need to adjust your dosage.

■ TESTOSTERONE

Testosterone is usually thought of as a male hormone, but women make and need it, too. This steroid hormone is made in the testicles and adrenal glands of men, and in the ovaries and adrenal glands of women. Even after menopause, a woman's adrenal glands continue to make testosterone. As with estrogen and progesterone, the body benefits in many ways when testosterone levels are optimal and in balance with other hormones. Testosterone increases libido (sexual desire and satisfaction), improves mood, lessens depression, preserves memory, maintains and promotes muscle mass and strength, decreases body fat, increases exercise tolerance, protects against cardiovascular disease, improves cholesterol, maintains bone density, prevents osteoporosis, prevents tendon and joint degeneration, and maintains skin tone.

Optimal levels of testosterone are much lower for women than they are for men. When it is in excess or when there is a shortage, however, uncomfortable symptoms and health risks appear.

Symptoms of Low Testosterone

Most women in their sixties have only half the testosterone they had prior to the age of forty. It's not surprising that a woman approaching or passing menopause may have symptoms of low testosterone. Other conditions and exposures can also cause decreased testosterone at other stages of life, including childbirth, endometriosis, chronic stress, and the use of certain drugs such as cancer therapies, birth control pills, and cholesterol-lowering statin drugs like Crestor and Lipitor.

In addition to the hot flashes and night sweats commonly associated with low testosterone, the following symptoms are typical of someone with decreased levels of this hormone. If you are experiencing more than half of these conditions, your system may be lacking testosterone:

- Aching joints or arthritis
- Decreased exercise tolerance
- Depression or anxiety
- High total cholesterol
- Increased fat mass
- Lack of energy
- Leaky bladder
- Less lean muscle mass
- Loss of sexual interest
- Memory loss
- Osteoporosis
- Painful intercourse
- Poor concentration
- Poor skin tone
- Sagging skin and eyelids
- Thinning and dry hair or dry skin
- Vaginal dryness
- Weight gain or difficulty losing weight

Of course, even if you notice a number of these symptoms, it is important to pinpoint the cause of low testosterone before attempting to fix the problem. Once you have done so, you may wish to boost your testosterone levels naturally, which can be done by eating a protein-rich diet, restricting your calorie intake, exercising (both weight-bearing and cardiovascular), getting eight hours of restful sleep each night, reducing stress, losing fat mass, and taking zinc supplements. If you already follow these healthy practices and still experience symptoms of decreased testosterone, and your levels have been confirmed, you may be a candidate for testosterone replacement therapy. (See page 92.)

Symptoms of High Testosterone

Some women naturally produce high amounts of testosterone, others taking testosterone replacements can overdo it, causing elevated levels. While these women may enjoy some benefits of high testosterone levels (for example, an enhanced libido), they may be unlucky in other respects. Of note, women with polycystic ovarian syndrome tend to have high levels of testosterone. PCOS is a common disorder in young women (under forty-five years of age) that is linked with facial hair, insulin resistance, midsection obesity, infertility, irregular periods, and the absence of breast development.

The body was designed to help balance its own hormones. In both men and women, excess testosterone levels can be directly converted into either estrogen or dihydrotestosterone (DHT). The path of conversion depends on your genes and your environment. If excess testosterone is converted into DHT, this can lead to facial hair, midsection weight gain, acne, low fertility, erratic periods, and male-pattern baldness. If a woman's body prefers to turn excess testosterone into estrogen, she may have an easier time transitioning through menopause.

The following symptoms are commonly associated with high levels of testosterone. If you have more than half of the symptoms on this list, you probably have an excess of this hormone:

- Abdominal weight gain
- Acne or oily skin
- Compulsive sexual appetite
- Decreased HDL
- Depression or anxiety
- Difficulty falling asleep
- Elevated estrogen levels
- Elevated sexual appetite
- Excessive energy
- Hair growth at application site (if supplementing with topical testosterone)
- Hair growth on chin or upper lip
- Increased muscle mass
- Increased size of clitoris
- Insulin resistance or type II diabetes
- Male-pattern baldness
- Overly assertive or aggressive
- Polycystic ovarian syndrome
- Salt and sugar cravings

Spironolactone, a diuretic medication commonly prescribed for heart failure, liver disease, and high blood pressure, can also treat facial hair and acne caused by too much testosterone. The typical starting dosage is 100 mg daily, and it may take six or more months to see improvement. Side effects include increased potassium levels, nausea, diarrhea, fatigue, headache, irregular or heavy menstrual bleeding, and estrogen dominance.

Cimetidine is a medication usually prescribed to treat stomach ulcers. It can be used to treat excess testosterone, but spironolactone is about 500 times stronger, so I don't usually waste time recommending this medication.

Saw palmetto lowers levels of DHT. Many studies have shown that it can shrink enlarged prostates in men, but there are none proving effectiveness of the supplement in women. Even so, many naturopathic doctors recommend this herb to women with facial hair, and often their patients remain on it because of their results. A starting dosage can be 160 mg daily.

Finasteride, like saw palmetto, has been found to be a viable treatment option for women with extra facial hair. The usual dosage is 5 mg daily. It is expensive, and its side effects may include decreased sex drive, dry skin, and birth defects.

Metformin, a diabetes medication, can also treat symptoms of excess testosterone (increased facial hair, thinning hair of the crown, dandruff, acne), especially in women who have PCOS. A typical dose is 500 mg three times daily. Side effects include diarrhea, nausea, upset stomach, and (rarely) low blood sugar.

Other treatment options to decrease excess testosterone levels include losing weight, eating a vegetarian diet, taking flaxseed, supplementing with ECGC (green tea's active ingredient), taking oral estrogens (not recommended), and making sure your progesterone level is optimal. Obviously, if the excess was caused by an over-supplementation of testosterone, then your provider would decrease the dosage and reevaluate in a month.

■ THYROID HORMONES

The thyroid gland produces hormones that control cell growth, protein synthesis, metabolism, and body temperature. Thyroid hormones also affect brain function, tissue repair, blood flow, sex drive, mood, and energy levels. There are two types of thyroid hormones: thyroxine (T_4) and triiodothyronine (T_3). T_4 is the inactive form of thyroid hormone and must be converted into T_3 before it is effective. Much of this conversion happens in every cell in the body.

T_4 accounts for 80 to 95 percent of thyroid hormones in the body, though T_3 is five times more active. Both hormones require the amino acid tyrosine and the chemical element iodine for production. Each day, the body makes 90 to 100 mcg of T_4, a portion of which is then converted into T_3. The brain senses the supply and demand for thyroid hormones and keeps the levels of T_4 and T_3 in balance by sending a thyroid-stimulating hormone (TSH) to the thyroid gland when it is time to make more.

A lack of thyroid hormone production results in a condition called hypothyroidism. This problem can be caused by genetic defects, a deficiency in the thyroid starting materials tyrosine or iodine, a lack of the 5'-deiodinase enzyme, toxin overload, auto-immune reactions, aging, or stress.

Symptoms of Low Thyroid Hormones

The following symptoms are typical of someone who is experiencing low thyroid hormones levels. If more than half of these conditions apply to you, you likely have a thyroid hormone imbalance:

- Chronic headaches
- Cold hands and feet or poor circulation
- Constipation
- Decreased libido
- Depression, agitation, anxiety, or mood swings
- Dry skin or brittle nails
- Excessive fatigue
- Greater susceptibility to colds
- Hair thinning or loss
- High blood pressure
- High cholesterol
- Impaired memory
- Inability to concentrate
- Infertility
- Insomnia
- Low body temperature and cold intolerance
- Menstrual pain or irregularities
- Muscle and joint pain
- Puffy eyelids, loss of outer brows
- Reduced heart rate
- Unexplained weight gain
- Water retention

Some people's hypothyroidism may fall under the radar because their lab tests don't reveal the issue. These people have what is called subclinical hypothyroidism, in which they experience many hypothyroid symptoms but their thyroid hormone levels aren't severe enough for a diagnosis of full-blown hypothyroidism. Others have what is known as functional hypothyroidism, in which their thyroid hormone levels are optimal but a malfunction in either metabolism or hormone binding causes symptoms of low thyroid hormones.

The Importance of Iodine and Tyrosine

As you will recall, hypothyroidism can occur if you don't consume enough of the amino acid tyrosine or the mineral iodine. Although tyrosine deficiency is very rare, it can be caused by a lack of high-protein foods (including soy, chicken, fish, lima beans, and peanuts) in the diet or a sluggish thyroid gland. In the unlikely event that tyrosine levels are low, supplementation can certainly help.

Contrary to popular belief, iodine deficiency still happens today, especially if you eat foods grown in iodine-deficient soil. The problem may also arise in reaction to iodine's competitors, the chemical compounds bromide and fluoride. Commercially baked goods generally contain bromide and tap water often has added fluoride. These substances disrupt iodine's role in thyroid hormone synthesis, rendering it inactive or hypoactive.

The iodine paint test is an easy way to tell if you are deficient in iodine. Start by painting a silver-dollar-sized area of iodine on the inside of your arm, leg, or abdomen. If the stain disappears completely within eight to ten hours, chances are you have an iodine deficiency. If this is the case, taking iodine supplements and avoiding bromide and fluoride sources can be effective ways to flush out iodine competitors and regain thyroid function without thyroid hormone supplementation.

Converting T_4 into T_3

As previously mentioned, the body makes two types of thyroid hormones: the hypoactive T_4, which has four iodine molecules, and the active T_3, which contains three iodine molecules. The thyroid gland, kidneys, liver, pituitary gland, and muscle tissues convert T_4 into T_3, aided by an enzyme called 5'-deiodinase, which removes one iodine molecule from T_4. If you don't have enough

Making and Transporting Steroid Hormones

Cholesterol is the starting ingredient for steroid hormones. These hormones can convert back and forth into each other depending on which one your body needs at the time. The conversions require enzymes, which are special proteins that help a biochemical reaction happen quickly. Many enzymes require vitamins to function properly, so if you are deficient in a certain vitamin, your hormones may become imbalanced.

of this enzyme, you may experience hypothyroid symptoms even if your T_4 levels are normal. This enzyme requires the mineral selenium to function. In addition, exposure to environmental pollutants such as PCBs, and heavy metals such as lead, mercury, cadmium, and arsenic, can interfere with this enzyme, preventing the conversion of T_4 into T_3.

To better visualize this principle, imagine your best friend knows how much you love her homemade vanilla walnut fudge. She heard from your husband that you're feeling down and wants to send you some. She whips up a batch, packages it, and sends it to you. You sign for the package and take it inside. But then you can't find your box cutter. Without the box cutter, all you have is a boring brown box that you can't open. You don't know what's in there, and you certainly can't taste what's inside.

A similar scenario can happen in your thyroid. Your brain senses that your body needs more thyroid hormone, so it sends thyroid-stimulating hormone. A functioning thyroid gland will whip up a batch of T_4, and a protein carrier will take that T_4 to cells throughout the body. Since cells needs thyroid hormones to maintain energy, they are happy to hear a knock at the door from T_4. But the body has not converted the hormone into the more active T_3 because it does not have the enzyme needed to do so. It's as though the body does not have a box cutter to get to the vanilla walnut fudge inside the box. Cells can have a stockpile of T_4, but not enough T_3, resulting in hypothyroidism.

Hypothyroidism can also occur when the body has too much of a hormone called reverse T_3 (rT_3). Because the body is designed to maintain hormonal balance, an enzyme called 5'-deiodinase can create reverse T_3 by removing a different iodine molecule from T_4. Reverse T_3 is the mirror image of T_3 (think of a left hand and a right hand) and has an anti-thyroid effect on the body. Basically, T_3 is the gas pedal and rT_3 is the brakes. Reverse T_3 can bind to and occupy a T_3 receptor and prevent T_3 from doing its job. While rT_3 is meant to restore balance to thyroid hormone levels, overproduction of this hormone will actually do the exact opposite. Whether you cannot maintain optimal amounts of T_3 or your rT_3 is too high, the imbalance will cause you to exhibit signs of hypothyroidism.

The fact is that you can experience hypothyroid symptoms even though your TSH and T_4 levels are normal. Many physicians test only for these substances, so your symptoms might not receive any further attention. If levels of T_3 are tested and found to be low, however, they may indicate that you are having trouble converting T_4 to T_3, or that 5'-deiodinase has become overactive and is creating reverse T_3. In either case, thyroid hormone supplementation (especially T_3) might be warranted. (See page 104.)

The Effect of Stress

Stress leads to high cortisol levels, which, in turn, depress thyroid-stimulating hormone in the brain. Cortisol also inhibits the conversion of T_4 to T_3 and lowers the function of thyroid receptors throughout the body. Conversely, low cortisol as seen in adrenal fatigue patients reduces the number of thyroid receptors inside cells. Adrenal fatigue patients who also have hypothyroidism should always correct their adrenal issues before fixing their thyroid problems.

Thyroid-binding Proteins

Over 99 percent of all thyroid hormones are attached to carrier proteins. Approximately 70 to 80 percent are bound to a protein called thyroxine-binding globulin (TBG), while much of the remainder is bound to a protein called albumin. These proteins help thyroid hormones travel throughout the body without being broken down. Only 0.4 percent of T_4 and 0.04 percent of T_3 are unbound. Unfortunately, only free T_4 and free T_3 can have any effect on the body. When they are bound to TBG or albumin, they cannot do their jobs.

Carrier proteins are necessary, of course, but sometimes too many of them can cause problems. For example, people who take birth control pills or oral estrogens can make too much TBG, which results in symptoms of hypothyroidism despite seemingly normal thyroid hormone levels. Even if you start supplementing with thyroid hormones, you may feel better at first, but in a few months time the signs of hypothyroidism will return, as TBG levels will have slowly crept up again. Therefore, it should be your clinician's aim to control TBG levels, probably by discontinuing oral estrogen therapy and cleaning out xenoestrogens from your system. (It should be noted that transdermal estrogen, or estrogen delivered through the skin, does not affect TBG levels, so if you need to supplement estrogen, your physician can switch your therapy to a topical cream or transdermal patch.)

Hashimoto's Thyroiditis

Another cause of hypothyroidism is the autoimmune disease Hashimoto's thyroiditis. Normally, a functioning immune system can distinguish self from non-self and only creates antibodies to memorize and attack foreign objects like viruses. In autoimmune diseases, however, the body sees an aspect of its own biology as a foreign intruder and mounts an attack on itself. In Hashimoto's thyroiditis, the body does not recognize the thyroid as part of itself and consequently, the immune system declares war on the thyroid gland and produces antibodies against it. Immune cells flock to the thyroid gland and start slowly destroying the tissue. Patients often feel discomfort in the neck, which may appear swollen, while levels of thyroid antibodies and the enzyme thyroid peroxidase (TPO) are elevated. Your hormone clinician should always check for thyroid antibodies and thyroid peroxidase as part of your hormone panel. Integrative physicians and naturopathic doctors are experienced in eliminating the cause of this autoimmune issue (often lifestyle related) and typically offer nutritional therapy along with thyroid supplementation as a means of treatment.

■ VITAMIN D

Maybe you are wondering what a vitamin is doing in the hormone section of this book. Maybe you're already aware of the trend of calling vitamin D "hormone D" instead. Vitamins must be ingested into the body, while hormones are produced in one part of the body and act on another part. According to this information, vitamin D is actually a hormone. Vitamin D is a fat-soluble substance that is activated within the skin upon the body's exposure to UVB rays of sunlight. It travels through your system telling cells to do tasks such as making certain proteins. Unlike other vitamins, vitamin D acts on cells in all tissues of the body and sends messages that influence genetic instruction. Over the last decade, numerous groundbreaking studies have been published about vitamin D and its amazing ability to reduce the risk of disease. It has been shown to protect against many illnesses, including osteoporosis, numerous forms of cancer (including breast cancer), cold and flu viruses, multiple sclerosis, diabetes, and heart disease.

Bone Health

Vitamin D encourages calcium absorption in the gut, helps maintain bone density, and is essential for building and repairing bone. For years, it has been known that vitamin D prevents rickets in children (soft bones, increased fractures, irregular development) and decreases the risk of osteoporosis later in life. In fact, vitamin D should always be a part of a healthy lifestyle because of its ability to maintain strong bones. Consider that vitamin D levels are consistently low in elderly people who fall and fracture their bones.

Cancer

If a cell divides over and over and never dies, it is considered cancerous. Vitamin D helps healthy cells maintain their lifecycles and die when it is time. Often a cancer cell will stimulate nearby blood vessels to grow, allowing a tumor to flourish. Vitamin D also helps prevent cells from taking over their environments, thus inhibiting tumor growth.

Flu

Vitamin D also fights the flu and the common cold. The Centers for Disease Control (CDC) reports that 5 to 20 percent of the population of the United States catches the flu every winter. Of those, 200,000 people are hospitalized and 36,000 die from it. As a result, the CDC recommends that 84 percent of the United States get vaccinated against the flu. Most flu vaccines, however, contain harmful substances such as mercury (thimerosal), formaldehyde, and aluminum. Thimerosal, which is 50 percent mercury by weight, is used to disinfect the vaccine. The mercury content in most vaccines contains 250 times more mercury than the Environmental Protection Agency's safety limit. Formaldehyde is used to inactivate the virus, but it is a known carcinogen. Aluminum is added to promote an antibody response, but it is a neurotoxin linked to Alzheimer's disease. Some other additives found in the flu vaccine are traces of chicken metabolites, Triton X-100 (a detergent), Polysorbate 80, carbolic acid, ethylene glycol (antifreeze), gelatin, and various antibiotics. All can cause allergic reactions in some people.

The flu virus exists in people year round, though epidemics occur during the cold part of the year. Explanations have included the closer contact people have with each other when indoors, the drier air that dehydrates mucus and keeps the body from expelling virus particles, and the longer life of a virus in a cold temperature. But this does not explain why flu epidemics also happen where the weather stays warm all year. In such places, these epidemics happen during the rainy season. The common factor, in fact, is a lack of sunlight. In the tropics, the rainy season brings thick rain clouds, and in temperate zones, the earth's atmosphere blocks most vitamin D-producing UVB rays during the winter. Also, skin is less exposed at this time. Flu season happens when people's vitamin D levels are at their lowest. Since vitamin D promotes the immune response, flu epidemics may actually be linked to vitamin D deficiency.

Inflammation

Vitamin D also inhibits and lessens inflammation, which is a contributor to many diseases. Vitamin D has been shown to decrease the inflammatory substance TNF-alpha (tumor necrosis factor-alpha). TNF-alpha is produced by white blood cells (the body's defenders) in response to an attack on the body. The result is inflammation, fever, increased cortisol, and decreased appetite. It's good that TNF-alpha stimulates the immune system to fight an acute attack, but ongoing inflammation can lead to disease (including cardiovascular disease). Inflammation can also turn the body against itself, as happens in rheumatoid arthritis, multiple sclerosis, and asthma. Lowering levels of TNF-alpha through vitamin D supplementation may improve these disease states.

Vitamin D Production

Regular exposure of skin to the sun allows the body to make vitamin D. If you bare your arms, legs, face, or back to sunlight for twenty to thirty minutes twice a week between the hours of 10 AM and 3 PM without wearing sunscreen, each session will yield 10,000 to 20,000 IU (International Units) of vitamin D. To get the maximum effect, however, you cannot wash your skin immediately after exposure—you need to wait up to ten hours before showering to properly absorb the vitamin D made! Vitamin D production can be reduced by half or even more by a variety of factors, including latitude, time of day, season, sunscreen, skin color, shaded areas, clouds, and pollution. Those living at latitudes north of Boston will not be able to obtain sufficient vitamin D synthesis from the sun from November through February. Those living farther north may not get proper sunlight for up to six months of the year. Conversely, those living along the southern California and South Carolina latitude can expect to make sufficient vitamin D throughout the year.

It's true that using sunscreen, wearing protective clothing, or staying in the shade while outdoors can prevent sunburns and skin cancer. But wearing any sunscreen with an SPF higher than 8, or staying completely covered in clothing or under shaded areas, will block vitamin D production. To get the best of both worlds, get your direct sunshine for fifteen minutes without sunblock, and then apply it if you wish to extend your time in the sun. Those with very pale skin, however, may not be able to bear

---

Risk Factors for Vitamin D Deficiency

- Aging skin (cannot synthesize vitamin D as efficiently)
- Consistent use of sunblock (blocks UVB light)
- Dark skin (blocks more UVB light than light-colored skin)
- Diet poor in vitamin D (lacks salmon or tuna, and fortified milk or cereal)
- No skin exposure to sun (from working indoors)
- Obesity (fat locks up vitamin D and varies its release into the blood)

such recommendations and should obtain vitamin D solely from diet and supplements. Conversely, African Americans or those with very dark skin, which naturally blocks sunlight absorption, may need five to ten times as much sun exposure as light-skinned people. Unfortunately, dark-skinned individuals have the greatest risk of vitamin D deficiency.

Vitamin D Supplementation

While vitamin D is not the focus of this book, its overall importance to the human body requires the inclusion of a brief word about supplementation. As the previously mentioned information suggests, many people may need to take a vitamin D supplement. There is evidence to suggest that the current Recommended Daily Intake of vitamin D, which is between 400 and 600 IU, is simply insufficient. Experts now advocate an optimal daily dosage of 2,000 to 5,000 IU for adults and 2,000 to 3,000 IU for teenagers. They also recommend supplementing with vitamin D_3, also known as cholecalciferol, instead of vitamin D_2, also known as ergocalciferol, as vitamin D_3 is the more effective form.

Ultimately, different people often require different dosages to achieve optimal health and disease prevention, so always consult your doctor to find out the right dosage for your body. Individuals who take vitamin D_3 at high dosages (more than 2,000 IU per day for adults) should have their blood vitamin D levels checked every six months to one year. Taking too much vitamin D can result in nausea, vomiting, decreased appetite, constipation, weight loss, and weakness. More serious health risks include changes in mental status, abnormal heart rhythm, and kidney stones. Typically no toxic effects are seen if serum levels remain below 200 ng/mL.

If you don't wish to take supplements, diet is another way to increase your vitamin D level. Fish has the highest natural content of this nutrient. Good sources are salmon, mackerel, sardines, and tuna, while cod liver oil is the most potent food source of vitamin

D. In addition, other foods are often fortified with vitamin D, including orange juice, milk, yogurt, and cereal.

HOW HORMONES AFFECT EACH OTHER

When a storm closes an airport, there are often delays at many other airports, even those far away. Since each airport has dozens or hundreds of flights, any delay or cancellation can affect flight plans with seemingly no direct connection. Your endocrine glands are like airports; what happens in one affects many others. For example, when the ovaries shut down during menopause and produce less estrogen, hormones with no obvious connection become unbalanced. The fact is that hormones affect each other directly and indirectly in many ways.

Progesterone and Estrogen

Estrogen has "connecting flights" with many hormones, especially progesterone. Estrogen and progesterone often affect the body in opposite ways. For example, estrogen decreases sex drive, causes bloating, and stimulates breast tissue; while progesterone restores sex drive, acts as a diuretic, and protects against fibrocystic breasts. Excessive amounts of one of these hormones can actually lower the number of receptors for the other. These sister hormones must be in perfect balance, or an excess of one can create a deficiency in the other.

Progesterone also affects estrogen by influencing the conversion of testosterone into estrogen. This action requires an enzyme called aromatase, which is typically abundant in fat tissue. Essentially, progesterone puts the brakes on the production of this enzyme. If progesterone is low, the brakes won't work very well, and testosterone will be easily converted into estrogen. In turn, estrogen levels will become too high, and testosterone can become depleted. On the other hand, when there is too much progesterone, it denies the conversion of testosterone into estrogen. This results in depleted estrogen and a buildup of testosterone.

Testosterone and Estrogen

Like progesterone and estrogen, testosterone and estrogen also have a teeter-totter relationship. The rate of conversion of testosterone into estrogen can cause excesses or deficiencies in either hormone. Thus, there is a very fine line between balanced and unbalanced. You can have perfectly normal levels of estrogen but still complain of symptoms of estrogen dominance, simply because your level of testosterone is low relative to estrogen.

An excess of an enzyme called 5-alpha-reductase can cause high levels of the type of testosterone known as DHT. The enzyme 5-alpha-reductase converts testosterone into DHT, which is twice as potent as testosterone and causes male sex characteristics. Thankfully, there are a number of ways to minimize DHT production, such as losing weight, eating a vegetarian diet, adding flaxseed to your meals, supplementing with ECGC (the active ingredient in green tea) and saw palmetto, making sure your progesterone is optimal, and, if all else fails, taking Proscar (a prescription 5-alpha-reductase blocker).

The delicate balance between testosterone and estrogen can also be affected by changes in sex hormone-binding globulin (SHBG), a protein that carries hormones through the blood. A hormone that is bound to SHBG cannot affect tissues in the body. During perimenopause, there is a decrease in SHBG, which, in turn, frees up more testosterone. This is one of the reasons that some women experience more sexual desire or activity at this time. Other factors that can lower SHBG are low thyroid hormone levels, high cortisol, obesity, and increased insulin.

Interestingly, women taking estrogen orally as hormone replacement therapy during menopause will often have an increase in SHBG, lowering the levels of free testosterone. This phenomenon, however, is not seen in transdermal estrogen therapy. Some other factors that increase SHBG are raised thyroid hormones, increased estrogen, smoking, caffeine intake, and a vegetarian diet.

Cortisol

Cortisol affects many other hormones. Unlike progesterone, cortisol puts the gas on the production of aromatase, speeding the conversion of testosterone into estrogen. During periods of chronic stress, therefore, estrogen levels rise (while testosterone may fall). If progesterone is also low during times of stress, estrogen accumulates even faster. Unfortunately, cortisol also affects progesterone. As cortisol increases, it tells the brain that the body is under stress. The brain then tells the ovaries to stop making progesterone. As such, estrogen dominance and some degree of infertility are often results of chronic stress.

A high level of cortisol also makes thyroid imbalances worse. For example, excess cortisol can cause protein carriers to bind to thyroid hormones. As you know, bound thyroid hormones do not have any effect on the body. Ultimately, this problem will lead to hypothyroid symptoms. In this case, getting the cortisol level under control will not only help your adrenal glands, but also get your thyroid function back on track.

The cortisol-thyroid relationship also goes in the opposite direction. The thyroid gland can increase the breakdown of cortisol. So, if you have both adrenal insufficiency (low cortisol) and hypothyroidism, the cortisol problem will get even worse if you treat the thyroid and not the adrenal glands.

Additionally, cortisol has a relationship with testosterone. Think of them as the cousins that never get along at family reunions. No matter what the topic of conversation, cortisol will always disagree with testosterone and vice versa. When testosterone tries to send a signal to a tissue in your body, any available cortisol will try to block the signal. This explains why some people have normal testosterone levels but still experience symptoms of low testosterone.

Thyroid Hormones

When estrogen is low, thyroid hormones have a stronger effect on the body. Conversely, when estrogen is high, hypothyroidism can occur. This is because excess estrogen can prevent the thyroid from working well. In turn, low thyroid function can affect estrogen. A low level of thyroid hormones can cause estrogen to break into a harmful xenoestrogen called 6-alpha-OH estrone.

Progesterone is another sex hormone with which the thyroid has a relationship. The active thyroid hormone, T_3, signals the ovaries to release progesterone. Thus, when the thyroid is overactive, progesterone levels are high and estrogen levels are low. Conversely, an underactive thyroid does not stimulate progesterone production, and this lack of progesterone leads to estrogen dominance.

Insulin

Insulin is the hormone in charge of moving excess glucose from

Prescription Drugs and Hormone Levels

Many prescription drugs alter hormone levels, throwing off the body's hormonal balance. For example, the antidepressant drugs known as selective serotonin reuptake inhibitors (SSRIs), including Prozac, Paxil, and Zoloft, tend to lower progesterone levels, which can make perimenopause worse. Additionally, birth control pills and the statin class of cholesterol-lowering drugs, such as Lipitor, Zocor, and Mevacor, tend to lower testosterone. In a more startling example, patients taking opiates chronically for pain will find that these drugs not only suppress endorphin production but also hormone production—specifically cortisol, DHEA, and estrogen in women, and testosterone in men. If you take prescription drugs, make sure to talk to your pharmacist or physician to see if these substances might be contributing to symptoms related to menopause.

the blood into tissues for later use. The form of estrogen called estradiol can help drive glucose into cells, and can even promote insulin secretion. So, during menopause, if you are told you are becoming insulin resistant, prediabetic, or diabetic, you may need estrogen replacement to help promote or restore your tissues' insulin sensitivity. In turn, insulin can affect estrogen levels. A high level of insulin can cause estrogen to soar.

Progesterone supplementation appears to alleviate the problems associated with high insulin levels and helps balance insulin and glucose levels. It does not worsen insulin resistance. Progesterone can also lower triglycerides and improve polycystic ovary syndrome (PCOS).

DHEA

DHEA affects virtually everything in the body. It is a hormone whose main function is to act as a reservoir for estrogen, progesterone, testosterone, and cortisol production. As mentioned earlier, DHEA is made in the adrenal glands and stored in fat cells. Athletes, or other individuals with a low percentage of body fat, tend to be deficient in DHEA, and therefore are often deficient in estrogen or other hormones.

It is very important to avoid both DHEA excess and deficiency. It must remain in balance. Too much DHEA may result in elevated testosterone or estrogen levels. On the other hand, aging and stress can deplete stores of DHEA, causing progesterone, testosterone, and estrogen levels to plummet and cortisol levels to soar. If you are considering taking DHEA as a supplement, have your hormone levels checked first.

CONCLUSION

As the previous information shows, hormones play a wide range of important roles in the body. From maintaining a lean physique and preserving a hearty sexual appetite to balancing mood and sharpening mental acuity, hormones are the centerpiece of total health and wellness. While each hormone has their own distinct functions, you will feel healthiest when they are all working togeth-er at their proper levels and in balance with each other. Unfortu-nately, hormones tend to decrease in amount or become unbalanced as you age, leaving you feeling sluggish and less fit. The trick to wellness may just be restoring your hormonal balance through the use of bioidentical hormone replacement therapy under the super-vision of your doctor.

2

Hormone
Replacement Therapy

It is likely that most women you know, at one point or another in their lives, have experienced some type of hormonal imbalance. It is also likely that they have sought some form of hormonal remedy for the issue. Understanding the hormonal changes that affect a woman throughout the various stages of life is helpful when confronted by typical perimenopausal and menopausal symptoms, which are due to hormonal fluctuations or imbalances. It can also help you learn if hormone replacement therapy is a viable option for your situation. But, as with many new treatments, there is controversy surrounding hormone replacement therapy. In short, some in the medical community feel that all hormone replacements are dangerous, while others say that there must be a distinction made between bioidentical replacements, which appear safe to use, and non-bioidentical replacements, which have been linked to negative side effects. Once you know the difference between these two forms of hormone replacement therapy, you will be better able to move forward confidently with your choice of treatment when faced with the symptoms of hormonal imbalance.

THE REPRODUCTIVE STAGES OF A WOMAN'S LIFE

Being able to recognize when and how a woman's body changes throughout her life will help you know what to expect during these transitions. During a particular stage, a woman may experience uncomfortable hormonal imbalances. It is perfectly normal for a woman to deal with monthly hormonal ebbs and flows during the child-bearing years of her adulthood. As menopause approaches, certain hormones plummet and others follow suit, leading to overall hormonal declines during the last half of adulthood. Many women function just fine with low to nonexistent hormone levels, while others have a hard time weathering the perimenopausal and menopausal storms. A little hormone replacement therapy can go a long way in making a mature woman feel healthy and vibrant again. While not all menopausal women require hormone replacement therapy, many of them can achieve wellness through the use of this treatment. In order to understand how certain hormone replacement regimens may be beneficial at certain points in a woman's life, you first need to become acquainted with these stages and the hormonal fluctuations that define them.

Premenopause

This stage starts at approximately twelve years of age with the first menstrual cycle and lasts until menses, or periods, become less frequent. During these years, the skin is toned and supple, the body is lean, and the body's metabolism is fully functioning. You may already know the basics of the menstrual cycle, but you may not know which hormones are responsible for which phases or physical effects. By appreciating this complicated process, you will become more aware of the hormonal changes that occur throughout adulthood.

The Menstrual Cycle: Days One to Seven (The Period)

On day one, the period starts, lasting an average of three to seven days. During this stage, the body expels the unfertilized egg and excess uterine lining that has formed in preparation for pregnancy.

The Menstrual Cycle:
Days Eight to Thirteen (Pre-Ovulation)

Toward the end of the period, the brain sends a hormone called follicle-stimulating hormone (FSH), which signals estrogen levels to rise. The elevated estrogen level in the body stimulates about ten eggs in the ovaries and prepares the uterus for pregnancy. When estrogen peaks, the most developed egg with the most receptors becomes the lucky chosen one to head down a fallopian tube during the next stage of menstruation, while the other candidates begin to waste away. The level of estrogen begins to taper slightly at this point.

The Menstrual Cycle:
Day Fourteen (Ovulation)

Ovulation is the day a woman's body releases its egg. The brain raises the level of luteinizing hormone (LH), which helps the egg break out of the ovary. The egg then travels down a fallopian tube to be fertilized. Progesterone levels begin to climb and basal body temperature rises by about 1°F.

The Menstrual Cycle:
Days Fifteen to Twenty-Eight (The Luteal Phase)

After ovulation, progesterone continues to rise sharply, while estrogen levels stay fairly strong. The elevated amount of progesterone thickens and seals the uterine lining that estrogen helped grow in preparation for pregnancy, allowing the egg to implant itself. The egg then awaits a sperm to fertilize it. After a few days of waiting to be fertilized, both estrogen and progesterone levels plummet. This fall of hormones triggers the menstrual period to shed the uterine lining. If the egg happens to get fertilized before these hormone levels drop, progesterone will stay high throughout pregnancy and the uterine lining will remain.

Perimenopause

When a woman is in her early twenties, all her hormones are at their peak levels. They then gradually decline, which leads to the next stage in reproductive life, called perimenopause. Perimenopause lasts about two to eight years. Women enter this transitional period between the ages of thirty-five and fifty-five, meaning half of a women's life may be spent after menopause. I wish women in our culture were given more guidance about this phase. Armed with the required knowledge, we might then be better prepared for this physical and emotional change.

Perimenopause is the transitional stage into menopause during which the ovaries start to run out of good eggs. In reaction, the brain starts sending either stronger or erratic amounts of FSH to the ovaries, thus yielding more eggs than usual and promoting pregnancy. This also results in increased and often fluctuating estrogen levels. At times, ovulation doesn't happen at all. During such cycles, progesterone never shows up, which causes symptoms of estrogen dominance, including bloating, irritability, weight gain, breast tenderness, headaches, and an overgrowth of the uterine lining. A woman may start spotting, bleed heavily for long periods of time, or skip her period entirely. Most women who experience these miserable symptoms can't put their finger on what is really happening. Serum blood tests are usually not useful, as they can give different results from day to day. A doctor may recommend an antidepressant for mood issues, birth control pills to normalize the menstrual cycle, and a weight-loss regimen to decrease other symptoms. These remedies are typically prescribed after a ten-minute medical exam. A better course of action, in my opinion, would be to find a provider who will take the time to explain this stage of life and all it entails. I wish more young women who experience signs of estrogen dominance or changes in their cycles would seek an experienced hormone specialist. Many thirty-something women don't realize that they have already entered perimenopause, and their problems do not receive proper treatment.

Menopause

According to the medical establishment, a woman can consider herself in menopause when she has gone twelve consecutive months without experiencing a menstrual period. During this year, ovarian function stops and both estrogen and progesterone levels plummet. This lack of estrogen and progesterone puts an end to menstrual cycles.

The average age of onset of menopause is fifty-one. In addition, the onset of menopause is influenced by genetics and environment. For example, smokers transition to menopause eighteen months sooner, on average, than non-smokers. Other conditions associated with earlier menopause include surviving a childhood cancer, having epilepsy, living at high altitudes, enduring economic hardship, and dealing with major depression. A woman can also be pushed into menopause overnight by the surgical removal of both ovaries. Women who experience early menopause may also have more severe symptoms.

Symptoms of Menopause

For many women, menopause can be accompanied by a myriad of symptoms felt from head to toe. Many of these conditions are due to the decreased production of estrogen, progesterone, and testosterone that characterizes menopause. While menopause (and perimenopause) can seem like a debilitating and unhealthy time in a woman's life, the truth is that most women will experience only a few of the following symptoms:

- **Hot flashes.** The hallmark symptom of menopause is hot flashes, which are typically caused by low estrogen and elevated FSH levels. A hot flash is the feeling of intense heat originating in the chest and rising up to the face or neck. The heat causes sweating and rapid heart rates, and can last from a few minutes up to half an hour. In severe cases, some women experience hot flashes every hour that can be felt throughout the entire body. Hot flashes can have a tremendously negative impact on quality of life and are often accompanied by anxiety and embarrassment.

- **Metabolic issues.** A lack of estrogen can make diabetes worse or promote insulin resistance. A lack of testosterone can cause fatigue, a reduction in muscle mass, and an increase in fat. Decreased progesterone can also cause weight gain.

- **Mood disturbances.** Many women report irritability, anxiety, depression, and difficulty concentrating, also known as brain fog. While various causes of these conditions are possible (for example, stress), hormonal changes are well known to influence mood.

- **Sleep disturbances.** Sleep can be disrupted by night sweats, which are hot flashes during sleep. Sleep can also be affected by a hormonal imbalance, such as progesterone insufficiency or a cortisol issue.

- **Vaginal atrophy and sexual problems.** Vaginal atrophy—the thinning and drying of the tissues in and around the vagina—can cause itching, burning, and discomfort during sexual intercourse. This, along with low testosterone levels, can contribute to sexual dysfunction and a lack of libido.

The frequency and severity of these conditions differ greatly from woman to woman. Why? Some women take care of themselves throughout their lives. They keep their waistlines in check, eat whole foods without preservatives and pesticides, never smoke, rarely drink, have a positive outlook on life, and embrace the support of their loved ones—all of which pays off during this transition. Other women are simply born with good genes that help their hormones remain in balance.

Postmenopause

Postmenopause is the phase after menopause. It starts between twenty-four and thirty-six months after a woman's final period and continues throughout the rest of her life. In this stage, a woman is no longer fertile. Unless obtained from external means such as hormone replacement therapy, hormone levels remain low or absent. Most women at this time of life, especially those long past menopause, don't consider hormone therapy, since their hot flashes and other severe menopausal symptoms have naturally subsided. After menopause, though, estrogen deficiency increases the risk of health problems such as the following:

- **Cardiovascular disease.** An increase in overall cholesterol and a decrease in HDL cholesterol raise the risk of cardiovascular disease. The changes may be indirectly linked to the fact that it is harder to maintain lean muscle mass and exercise after menopause.

- **Musculoskeletal issues.** Numerous studies have found a much greater risk of bone fracture and osteoporosis after menopause. This is important because falls and fractures are a major cause of death in the elderly. Arthritis is another disease often considered just part of growing old, but progesterone and testosterone insufficiencies can make arthritis worse. Shrinking muscles due to low testosterone levels may be the main reason for bone loss and achy joints.

Women may also experience thinning scalp hair or a few facial whiskers during this period. Additionally, the wrinkles, fine lines, and sagging and dry skin that are normally associated with aging become worse after menopause.

Reclaiming Your Life

It is unfortunate that once your hormones stop working for you, so do many other parts of your body. Joints, bones, cardiovascular system, skin, hair, mood, cognition, and so on may start to give you problems. By comparing photos taken before menopause and about a year after menopause, the unflattering effects on the appearance and health status of an individual are noticeable.

If left untreated, these issues grow worse over time. If you take care of yourself and balance your hormones, however, you can still have mounds of energy, a hearty sexual appetite, a trim waistline, and a zest for life. As a bonus, you will also find yourself wiser and more confident than when you were younger. (You also won't have to worry about periods or birth control anymore!)

The fact is that you don't have to suffer through the health conditions brought about by hormonal changes anymore. Starting now, you can change your lifestyle and balance your hormones with hormone replacement therapy. The first step on the road to reclaiming your well-being is to understand the controversy surrounding HRT and the way in which bioidentical hormone replacement therapy (BHRT) is different.

THE HORMONE REPLACEMENT CONTROVERSY

When discussing hormone replacement therapy, it is important to classify whether the hormones being taken are bioidentical or not. Bioidentical hormones—also known as human-identical hormones—have the exact chemical structure as hormones produced by the human body and will fully replicate all the functions of regular hormones. The body cannot tell the difference between a bioidentical hormone supplemented from the outside world and the hormone it makes on its own. Most pharmaceutical-grade bioidentical hormones start with materials such as yam or soy (substances that are natural but not bioidentical), which are then transformed in the laboratory into human-identical hormones. After this conversion, there is no trace of the yam or soy plant left. Examples of bioidentical hormones are compounded estriol cream and progesterone vaginal suppositories.

In contrast, many hormone replacement supplements are artificial. Created in a lab, these substances are not found in nature and have different structures than hormones made by the human body, making them non-bioidentical. They can still attach to hormone receptors and communicate messages to cells, but those messages may not be exactly like the ones produced by regular hormones. In fact, artificial hormones can give the opposite instructions, causing side effects or even promoting disease. Because its structure does not identically match that of the hormone it seeks to replace in the human body, this type of hormone replacement is not an ideal therapy option. Examples of these supplements include methyltestosterone (Android) and medroxyprogesterone (Provera).

Additionally, other hormones used in HRT are called "natural" because they come directly from nature and are not altered in any manner. The fact that these substances are not artificial, however, does not mean they are identical to the hormones made by the human body. For example, the hormone replacement Premarin is composed of estrogens extracted from a pregnant horse's urine. These estrogens can be considered natural, since they are taken from a source that naturally produces the hormone and unaltered, but they are not identical to human estrogens. Therefore, even though a product claims to be natural, it might not be bioidentical. I don't know about you, but I don't want to put horse urine in my body, even if it is natural. In addition, the estrogens in Premarin are literally built for a horse and thus are much more potent than those produced by women, which can lead to problems. While it may sound ideal, a natural source of hormones is not necessarily best for hormone replacement therapy.

So, why aren't all hormone replacement supplements bioidentical? The answer is that most pharmaceutical companies aren't interested in producing human-identical hormones, as there is little profit in doing so. These corporations make their money from drugs that can be patented, giving themselves exclusive manufacturing rights, profits, and privileges for many years. They can't patent bioidentical hormones, so instead they create drugs that attempt to mimic the activities of human hormones. For instance, drug companies can take human-identical progesterone, slightly alter its chemical structure, and *voilà:* They've created a patentable and profitable drug (for example, Provera) that is similar but not identical to the human hormone. The unfortunate consequence of this practice is that consumers get overcharged for a wannabe hormone that isn't any safer than the real thing and may even lead to a number of serious health conditions, including cancer. A closer look at non-bioidentical sex hormone replacements reveals their problems.

Non-Bioidentical Testosterone

For years, supplemental testosterone had to be injected or taken as an oral tablet, which was poorly absorbed. To get around these problems, drug manufacturers in the 1950s developed artificial versions of testosterone that could be better absorbed orally. But convenience came at a price. Artificial testosterone such as methyltestosterone (Testred, Halotestin) has a different pharmaceutical profile than bioidentical testosterone and has been associated with the following adverse reactions in women:

- **Cardiovascular.** Increased risk of bleeding in patients who take blood thinners, and raised cholesterol.

- **Dermatological.** Facial hair, male-pattern baldness, and acne.

- **Gastrointestinal.** Nausea, jaundice, altered liver function, abnormal liver cell growth, and abnormal blood cavities in the liver.

- **Genitourinary.** Irregular or cessation of periods, deepening of the voice, irreversible clitoral enlargement. When administered to a pregnant woman, causes changes to the external genitalia of the female fetus.

- **Neurological.** Increased or decreased libido, headache, anxiety, depression, and generalized numbness.

Other side effects include disturbances in the body's electrolyte balance such as the retention of sodium, chloride, water, potassium, calcium, and inorganic phosphates.

Non-Bioidentical Progesterone

Progestins are the synthetic progesterone-like compounds found in birth control pills and conventional hormone replacement therapies. Progestins like medroxyprogesterone acetate (Provera) are often prescribed to replace progesterone. Provera is similar in structure to progesterone and can bind to and act on the human progesterone receptor, but it is not identical to progesterone. As a result, it can produce physiological effects that progesterone does not. Hence, a woman taking Provera may experience insomnia, whereas a woman taking bioidentical progesterone will have restful sleep. Since progesterone receptors are found from head to toe, a woman who takes non-bioidentical progesterone may feel its unnatural effects throughout her entire body.

A number of studies have shown that progestins increase the risk of developing breast cancer, heart attacks, strokes, dementia, and blood clots. Moreover, other studies have not found an association between these health concerns and bioidentical progesterone. If you are thinking about trying a progestin or even a progestogen (a combination of bioidentical progesterone and a progestin) as hormone replacement therapy, you may want to reconsider. The following adverse reactions have been reported in connection with these types of treatment:

- **Breast.** Tenderness or pain, and spontaneous milk flow.

- **Cardiovascular.** Blood-clotting disorders, vein inflammation related to a blood clot, and blood clots in the lungs.

- **Dermatological.** Hives, itching, swelling, rash, acne, thinning scalp hair, and increased facial hair.

- **Gastrointestinal.** Nausea and jaundice.

- **Genitourinary.** Abnormal uterine bleeding (irregular, increased, or decreased), change in menstrual flow, breakthrough bleeding, spotting, absent menstrual period, and changes in cervical secretions.

- **Neurological.** Depression, insomnia, drowsiness, dizziness, headache, and nervousness.

- **Ocular.** Eye nerve lesions, retinal blood clots, and inflammation of the optic nerve.

Progestins have also been known to cause life-threatening allergic reactions, facial swelling, allergic rash (with or without itching), fever, fluid retention, fatigue, weight gain or loss, and decreased glucose tolerance, which can lead to diabetes.

Provera is the most common synthetic progestin used to treat symptoms of menopause. As previously mentioned, progestins are also found in many hormonal contraceptives, which sexually active women use to prevent pregnancy (Depo-Provera, Mirena, Alesse, Yasmin, YAZ, Ortho Tricyclen, Ortho-Novum, Enovid, Implanon, and Plan B). Women who take these contraceptives, therefore, may experience these side effects as well.

Non-Bioidentical Estrogens

One of the most popular estrogen replacement prescriptions for the treatment of menopause is Premarin. If you break apart its name, you will never forget how this product is made: Pregnant Mare's Urine. About 50 percent of estrogens in Premarin are termed conjugated equine estrogens (CEE) because they are identical to the horse estrogens equilin and equilenin. These equine estrogens have been associated with adverse reactions in the following areas:

- **Breast.** Tenderness, enlargement, pain, discharge, spontaneous flow of milk from the breast, fibrocystic or lumpy breasts (benign tumors), and an increased risk of breast cancer (according to the National Institutes of Health).

- **Cardiovascular.** Blood clots in the lungs or veins, vein inflammation, heart attack, stroke, and increased blood pressure.

- **Dermatological.** Darkening of facial skin that may persist after the drug is discontinued, mild or severe itchy rash that is red and symmetrical, inflammation of fat cells under the skin, severe blister-like rash, unwanted facial hair, loss of scalp hair, and itchy skin.

- **Gastrointestinal.** Nausea, vomiting, abdominal cramps, bloating, jaundice, gallbladder disease, inflammation of the pancreas, inflammation of and injury to the large intestine, and enlargement of non-cancerous liver tumors.

- **Genitourinary.** Abnormal uterine bleeding or spotting, severe uterine or pelvic pain during periods, inflammation of the vagina, bacterial or yeast vaginal infections, change in amount of cervical secretion, ovarian cancer, endometrial hyperplasia (excessive cell growth of the uterine lining), and endometrial cancer.

- **Neurological.** Headache, migraine, dizziness, depression, worsening of chorea (involuntary movement disorder), nervousness, mood disturbances, irritability, worsening of epilepsy, and dementia.

- **Ocular.** Retinal blood clots and intolerance to contact lenses.

Other problems linked to these hormones include diabetes, bloating, painful joints, leg cramps, changes in libido, hives, facial swelling, life-threatening allergic reaction, low calcium, worsening of asthma, elevated triglycerides, and an increase or decrease in weight. Although the other 50 percent of Premarin is composed of bioidentical estrogen, it is in the form of estrone, which has also been linked with an increased risk of developing breast cancer.

While all the previously mentioned side effects of traditional HRT are troubling, it is the connection with cancer (particularly breast cancer) that raises the most concern. But what exactly are the risks? And with which types of hormone replacement are these risks specifically associated?

Hormone Replacement Therapy and Breast Cancer

Prior to 2002, the estrogen supplement Premarin was the second most frequently prescribed medication in the United States. Millions of women were on hormone replacement therapy to treat the symptoms of menopause. In that same year, a study was released that caused many doctors to take their patients off HRT. It linked the practice to a number of serious health conditions, not the least of which was breast cancer. Other research that associated HRT with cancer soon followed. But what exactly do these studies mean? And do they apply to bioidentical hormone replacement therapy as well as non-bioidentical supplements like Premarin? The answers to these questions require a detailed look at the research.

Women's Health Initiative

The US government's National Institutes of Health conducted landmark research known as the "Women's Health Initiative" (WHI) in 2002. It compared the hormonal therapies Premarin (0.625 mg) and Provera (2.5 mg) with a placebo. The trial was fairly large, with more than 8,000 participants. The average age of the subjects was sixty-three, and the therapies were randomly assigned. Unfortunately, about 35 percent of volunteers dropped out of the study before it was completed—a fact that decreased the statistical significance of the findings. Even so, after more than five years, researchers discovered too many negative and alarming results associated with the hormonal therapies, causing them to stop the study. In summary, the results showed that Premarin and Provera, when taken together, increased a woman's risk of heart disease, stroke, blood clots, colon and breast cancers, fracture, and death. Premarin taken alone also promoted these risks, though not the incidence of breast cancer.

The Million Women Study

"The Million Women Study," which followed more than 1 million UK women between the ages of fifty and sixty-four from 1996 to 2001, published its results in 2003. The women were classified as either past or current users of hormone replacements for the treatment of menopausal symptoms. The women were separated into three groups: estrogen-only users, estrogen-plus-progestins users, and tibolone (a non-estrogen, non-progestin steroid hormone) users. No participants used or had used bioidentical progesterone. According to the study's findings, the individuals who used hormone replacement therapy during the research period showed a higher incidence of breast cancer. Furthermore, estrogen-plus-progestins therapy substantially increased the risk of breast cancer in comparison with the estrogen-only group, although the estrogen-only group still displayed an elevated risk of the disease.

It should be emphasized that the estrogen-only group of the "Million Women Study" took both natural and synthetic estrogen preparations, and that the level of dose made no difference to the outcomes. This means that if you decide to start using bioidentical estrogens alone, you should be mindful about the increased risk of breast cancer, regardless of your dosage.

Progesterone vs. Progestins

Led by Dr. Agnes Fournier, a study called "Breast Cancer Risk in Relation to Different Types of Hormone Replacement Therapy in the E3N-EPIC Cohort" looked at data on women who had used various hormone therapies from 1990 to 2002 to see whether the different types of progestagens used in HRT had produced different effects. It found that women who had taken estrogen together with progesterone showed no or slight increases in breast cancer when compared with women who had not received hormone therapy. Therefore, if you need to take hormones during menopause, you may be able to prevent the increased risk of breast cancer associated with supplemental estrogen by balancing this hormone with bioidentical progesterone (not synthetic progestins).

To further support Fournier's results, in 2005, Carlo Campagnoli and his colleagues reviewed numerous studies published in the United States and Europe on the risk of breast cancer in connection with HRT. According to their consensus, combined estrogen-progestin HRT increases the risk of breast cancer in comparison with estrogen-only regimens. Progesterone, however, does not increase the risk of breast cancer.

The E3N Study

Another study by Dr. Agnes Fournier ("Unequal Risks for Breast Cancer Associated with Different Hormone Replacement Therapies: Results from the E3N Cohort Study") examined data that was similar to her previously mentioned research. It found that the risk of breast cancer actually decreased when women were given weak estrogens, namely estriol and non-systemic vaginal estrogen preparations.

DeLignières French Cohort Study

This trial ("Combined HRT and Breast Cancer in French Women") followed more than 3,000 postmenopausal women for almost nine years, 55 percent of which had used some type of estrogen replacement therapy. Of the estrogen users, 83 percent had treated themselves with transdermal estrogen preparations and oral progesterone. The research found no increased risk of breast cancer among the women who had taken these hormones. The study's authors also noted that the women who had used topical estrogen did not have as many xenoestrogen metabolites as the women who had used oral estrogen. It is interesting to mention that most French women who take hormones use topical bioidentical estrogen preparations, and that there was no increased risk of breast cancer in this group according to this study.

Estriol Study

In 1966, a study led by Dr. Henry Lemon, a professor at the University of Nebraska, showed that women with high levels of estriol in their urine had a lower rate of breast cancer. Dr. Lemon followed up with an animal study, which found that rats that had been bioidentically pretreated with estriol before exposure to carcinogens were protected against breast cancer. (Estriol did, however, cause a growth of breast or uterine tissue in the rats.)

In 1977, Dr. Lemon did a clinical trail of estriol on women who already had breast cancer. Subjects received 2.5 to 5 mg per day of estriol therapy. There were twenty-eight premenopausal and postmenopausal breast cancer patients in the study. Estriol either induced remission or stopped growth of metastatic tumors in 37 percent of the women. These results suggest that estriol may be a good choice as HRT for breast cancer survivors experiencing symptoms of menopause.

The PEPI Trial

High breast density is a risk factor in the development of breast cancer. The "PEPI (Preoperative Endocrine Prognostic Index) Trial" was a large double-blinded placebo controlled study that looked at changes in breast density as a result of taking a placebo, conjugated equine estrogens (CEE) only, CEE and medroxyprogesterone (MPA), or CEE with progesterone therapies. The best feature of this large study is that it compared progestins with bioidentical progesterone therapy and analyzed their effects on breast tissue density. The results showed that estrogen has only a slight tendency to increase breast density, but when it is combined with a synthetic progestin (medroxyprogesterone acetate), breast density increases dramatically in the first year of HRT use. The risk of increased breast density when estrogen is combined with progesterone, however, was shown to be lower than with estrogen-progestin regimens, although it was still higher than the risk associated with estrogen-only therapy.

Hormone Profiles of Women with Breast Cancer

What do most women with breast cancer have in common? Dr. Barnett Zumoff can tell you. His study in 1994 revealed the typical hormonal profile of those who have this disease. In short, these women were found to have a decrease in the amount of androgens (testosterone and DHEA) being made in the adrenals, a certain ovarian dysfunction during the luteal phase (days 14 to 28) of the menstrual cycle, the tendency to generate xenoestrogen (specifically, an increase in 16 alpha-hydroxylation of estradiol), and a high level of the hormone prolactin.

Testosterone Studies

Testosterone's connection with breast cancer has been studied extensively—and the results are positive when it comes to its bioidentical form. The consensus of countless trials is that bioidentical testosterone inhibits the proliferation of breast cancer cells by possibly counteracting the stimulatory growth effects of estrogen. A notable study lead by Constantine Dimitrakakis in 2004 showed that adding testosterone to an estrogen or combined estrogen-progestin regimen may actually reduce the incidence of breast cancer.

Hormone Replacement Therapy and Other Cancers

Various other studies have reported that estrogen replacement therapy, whether bioidentical or not, increases the risk of endometrial cancer. Research has also shown, however, that pairing estrogen with either progesterone or a progestin decreases this risk. Therefore, it is standard practice that women (those who still have a uterus) who receive estrogen replacement therapy also take a form of progesterone to protect them from endometrial cancer. I recommend taking bioidentical progesterone. Those who use a progestogen cyclically won't have as much protection as those who receive it daily.

Women who follow this regimen should have an annual pelvic exam and see a doctor if unscheduled uterine bleeding occurs. Survivors of Stage I (beginning stage) endometrial cancer may still opt for hormones to treat menopausal symptoms as long as the estrogen is paired with some form of progesterone.

Although birth control pills containing both synthetic estrogens and progestins have been shown to reduce the risk of ovarian cancer by 50 percent, other studies have reported that postmenopausal women who use estrogen or a combination of estrogen and progestogen have a slightly increased risk of ovarian cancer. The risk becomes greater if women take hormone replacement therapy for more than ten years or at higher doses than normally prescribed. The general consensus among health professionals is that the risk of ovarian cancer due to hormone replacement therapy (whether bioidentical or non-bioidentical, estrogen-only or combined) is small and clinically insignificant.

Very few studies have found a connection between hormone replacement therapy and cervical cancer. Most cervical cancer cases are linked to the human papillomavirus (HPV), which is spread via unprotected sex. Estrogen-only replacement therapy may promote cervical cancer, but the evidence is weak.

Combination estrogen-progestogen replacement therapy has been shown to decrease the risk of colorectal cancer by one-third. Additionally, the WHI found no increase in risk of this type of cancer among women who used conjugated estrogens such as Premarin.

Finally, while artificial hormones do not seem to raise the risk of lung cancer, they do increase the rate of death from the disease.

Cancer Prevention

After all this talk about cancer, prevention must not be overlooked. Cancer happens when a cell starts to multiply itself uncontrollably. Exposures to toxins or infections, stress, lack of nutrients, a poorly functioning immune system, genetic mutations, and hormonal imbalance may each be linked to the disease. Breast cancer is often a result of hormonal imbalance and typically occurs after menopause, when your hormones are not within optimal range. You may minimize your risk of cancer by checking your hormone levels, using the lowest effective HRT doses and the proper routes of administration, supplementing with DIM, exercising regularly, eating organic foods, avoiding pesticides and chemicals, increasing your intake of omega-3 fatty acids, lowering your intake of omega-6 fatty acids, keeping overall dietary fat intake to less than 20 percent of total calories per day, increasing fiber intake to 45 g per day, limiting tobacco and alcohol consumption, checking for breast masses with thermography (not X-rays), and taking vitamins A, B, C, D, and E.

There is no research, however, on any connection between bioidentical hormones and lung cancer.

What the Research Tells Us

Unfortunately, most research on the relationship between hormone therapy and cancer is not divided neatly into a bioidentical hormone pile and a non-bioidentical hormone pile. The findings of some studies have caused health professionals to draw conclusions about all forms of hormone therapy, even if these findings do not apply to both bioidentical and non-bioidentical supplements. For example, the "Women's Health Initiative," which discovered the dangers of HRT, used conjugated equine estrogens (Premarin) and medroxyprogesterone acetate (Provera) in its trials. Although the findings of the WHI were not based on bioidentical hormones, they nevertheless discouraged physicians from prescribing any type of hormone replacement.

Alarm bells shouldn't sound when you hear the term bioidentical hormone replacement therapy. Estrogen and progesterone don't always have to be off-limits when it comes to your medicine cabinet. Are bioidentical hormones right for everyone? No. But certain types of bioidentical hormones may help many women with the symptoms of hormonal change while avoiding the negative health conditions associated with other forms of HRT. In some cases, bioidentical hormones may even be protective against disease. By digging a little deeper into the research, you may find that bioidentical hormone replacement therapy is right for you. There are always risks with any form of HRT, even bioidentical, but by learning more about this treatment option and speaking to your physician about your concerns, you may find a way to bring your system back into balance.

THE BIOIDENTICAL DIFFERENCE

Although the Food and Drug Administration (FDA) and the Endocrine Society have both stated that there is currently no evidence to support the effectiveness or safety of bioidentical hormone replacement therapy, Dr. Kent Holtorf of Holtorf Medical Group has compiled nearly 200 peer-reviewed papers describing the effectiveness and relative safety of bioidentical hormone therapy regimens (progesterone, estradiol, and estriol) versus synthetic hormone regimens (progestins and conjugated equine estrogens) in the treatment of menopause. After citing and analyzing various positive clinical outcomes of bioidentical hormone therapy, he concluded that bioidentical hormones are both safer and more effective than synthetic hormones and are the preferred method of hormone replacement therapy.

Hundreds of studies (many European) support the conclusion that BHRT is a reasonable therapeutic option for the treatment and relief of the many conditions associated with menopause. Many community health providers, unfortunately, still aren't well-versed in this subject. This fact may be due to the large amount of confusion surrounding BHRT. I believe that the drug industry and its practices are behind much of the confusion. To make a truly informed decision, you need to educate yourself on all the options, and pass the information on to your health care provider, if necessary.

Interpreting Studies

Some traditional doctors are skeptical of the current available research on bioidentical hormones. This may be because some of the studies citing positive results were small (not many patients enrolled), not double-blind to account for bias, and performed in Europe, where they may have less rigorous requirements for publication in a proper medical journal. Health professionals in the United States are taught to rely on large, double-blind, placebo-controlled trials (as required for FDA approval of drugs in the United States) to guide them in treatment options. Consider, though, that most drug research is funded and promoted by the manufacturer of the drug. Since bioidentical hormone therapy cannot be patented, there may never be a large, controlled study of this type of treatment.

Adding to the confusion, some prominent leaders in the United States health care system have made misleading statements about hormone research. For example, the primary investigator of the WHI, Dr. Jacques Rossouw, said in 2007, "The risks and benefits of all estrogens and all progesterones are equivalent." As you know, the WHI study involved only synthetic progestins (Provera) and horse estrogens (Premarin). If investigators want to lump all hormones together, they should perform studies that include bioidentical hormones too. In addition, Dr. Robert Vigersky of the American Medical Association has stated, "But there's no evidence that bioidenticals are any safer and they may even have other risks." No wonder providers are confused!

Drug Reps

Through sales calls made by drug representatives, many practitioners receive compelling information that a certain drug has an edge over another in the same class. While sometimes this is true, other times the information is simply a marketing tool to talk the doctor into prescribing that particular product. For example, after the WHI study showed the harmful effects of Premarin, the manufacturer of this drug made a new, low-dosage version and marketed it to doctors as a safer alternative. The marketing spin was that this lower dosage would be safer, since the higher amount of Premarin increased the risks of breast cancer and cardiovascular disease. There was, however, no actual evidence of improved safety associated with this lower dosage.

Some physicians are not particularly fond of prescribing the commercially available hormone products. But drug reps are consistently providing them with new studies about their products, as well as free samples to share with their patients. Meanwhile, compounding pharmacists and pharmacy reps do not heavily market bioidentical products. As a result, some doctors may not know that other options exist.

Resources for Your Health Provider

For a number for reasons, your health provider may not be comfortable prescribing bioidentical hormone replacements. She may be ignorant of them, skeptical of current bioidentical hormone research, or simply more familiar with traditional HRT. In the latter case, you may want to provide information about bioidentical hormones to your physician. You can share this book or a number of other books and journal articles on BHRT with her. A few notable web sites that may be helpful to your provider are www.worldhealth.net, www.functionalmedicine.org, and www.theifim.com.

Doctors who are open to bioidentical hormones but don't know where to begin often call pharmacists to ask about treatment options, risks, and starting dosages. Encourage your clinician to do the same. (Go to www.iacprx.org or www.pccarx.com for a compounding pharmacy referral).

Across the country, there are compounding pharmacies that prepare bioidentical hormone products customized for each patient. This offers physicians options in both dosages and formulations (creams or sublingual drops), as well as the ability to exclude preservatives, dyes, or allergens. The bioidentical hormones are prepared when the pharmacy receives the prescription, and most formulations expire in six months. Tailoring therapy to a patient's individual needs is important. Hormones should be given in the lowest effective dosages, each hormone supplemented should support hormonal balance, and personal risks and benefits should be discussed with a health care provider.

If your doctor is still unwilling to prescribe bioidentical hormone replacement therapy, go to www.bhrtsolutions.com to find an experienced physician. Of note, the American Academy of Anti-Aging Medicine (www.worldhealth.net), or A4M, is a non-profit organization dedicated to the advancement of technology that can detect, prevent, and treat age-related disease, and the promotion of research on how to slow the aging process. The A4M is also dedicated to educating physicians, scientists, and members of the public on biomedical sciences, breaking technologies, and anti-aging issues. The A4M offers a fellowship program in anti-aging and regenerative medicine, while the Institute for Integrative Medicine (www.theifim.com) offers a fellowship program in integrative and functional medicine.

CONCLUSION

Now you have an idea of which life stage you are in and what your hormonal profile probably looks like at this very moment—menopausal women have low hormone levels across the board and perimenopausal women have erratically fluctuating levels of estrogen and plummeting progesterone levels. It is imperative to get your doctor on board with how you want to handle your hormonal health situation. By understanding the controversy surrounding hormone replacement therapy, you are better equipped to find the right provider for your situation or prompt your current doctor to get educated. The next steps involve deciding if hormone replacement therapy is right for you and having your doctor design a hormone plan that includes a healthy lifestyle that promotes proper hormone receptor function and overall wellness.

3

Bioidentical Hormone Replacement Therapy Guidelines

enerally, individuals with low hormone levels, such as women going through menopause, may benefit from bioidentical hormone replacement therapy, but risks must be weighed against potential rewards. The decision to undergo treatment is typically based on the severity of symptoms, but every person is different and every situation is unique. There is no one-size-fits-all approach to BHRT, and no standard protocol of care. Since there is no agreed-upon protocol for treating hormonal imbalance with bioidentical hormones, it is impossible to recommend exact dosages of hormone replacements that would work for every person. The possibilities are infinite. Nevertheless, I can share treatment guidelines and dosage ranges based on my own clinical experience as well as the extensive experience of colleagues.

The best way to start bioidentical hormone replacement therapy is to take very low dosages, increasing them slowly over time until you achieve the optimal effect. Remember, everyone is unique, so amounts will vary. Your treatment must be determined by your hormone levels, symptoms, clinical situation, and goals. Therefore, it is imperative that you see an experienced HRT practitioner before starting therapy.

In addition, you may have to go beyond commercially available products to achieve your ideal hormonal balance. For example, the oral progesterone Prometrium is available only in 100-mg or 200-mg doses. Think of this issue as a shoe available in only two sizes. If your shoe size is 8, and the shoe store has only sizes 6 and 10, then the shoes there won't fit you, even if they are the cutest you ever saw. The size 6 will be too tight and the size 10 will just keep slipping off. Either way, you'll be miserable. Much like the shoes you wear, your dosages need to be the right "size" in order to make you comfortable. Thankfully, compounding pharmacies can make preparations that are right for your body.

USE CAUTION

Hormone replacement can be a valuable therapy for many women, but it carries serious risks that should be discussed with a physician. While I can share guidelines and insights into the way some of the top hormone experts make clinical decisions, it is not my intention that you make decisions without first consulting a health care provider or expert. If there were a cut-and-dried method to BHRT, then there wouldn't be so much confusion about the practice in the first place. Do not abuse this information. And do not take lightly the serious effects that hormones can have on your health.

While hormones can promote health and wellness, they are still powerful biochemical substances that can turn on or off all kinds of genes and proteins. Since the risk of many diseases and cancers increases with age, I typically steer women over sixty-five away from starting hormone replacement for the first time. So if, for example, you reached menopause at fifty-two and are now considering hormone therapy for the first time at age seventy-two, it may be best to use lifestyle changes, nutritional supplements, and certain herbs as the foundation of your plan to balance your hormone levels.

Women who take hormones are strongly urged to have an annual mammogram and cervical Pap smear. Even better is a thermogram or Halo breast Pap test; both are screening tools that assess a woman's future risk of breast cancer and do not use X-rays to do so. Conversely, a mammogram detects masses that may have already been growing for five years and uses X-rays (a type of ionizing radiation that can damage DNA and lead to cancer) to take a picture of the breast.

Some women should probably consider other treatments for their perimenopausal or menopausal symptoms. Consider alternatives if you have breast cancer (especially the type that is estrogen-receptor positive), unexplained genital bleeding, liver disease, are prone to blood clots, or are pregnant. (See "Alternatives to Hormone Replacement Therapy" on page 113.)

Hormone replacement at this time is a very sensitive subject with some traditional physicians because of the many conflicting literature references. You will need to educate yourself—and sometimes your doctor as well—to optimize your therapy and goals. Individuals who are not willing to challenge their health providers will probably have to seek therapy options other than bioidentical hormones.

GET DOSAGES RIGHT

Now that you know what hormones are, how and why your body uses and needs them, how they are related to each other, and what happens when one is out of balance, it makes sense to find out how to give your body back exact replicas of the hormones affected by menopause. Furthermore, not only do glands produce fewer hormones with age, but cells become less receptive to these substances. Fortunately, bringing hormones to their optimal levels and leading a healthier lifestyle increases receptor activity. It's extremely important, however, to give back only what your body needs, and give it back in perfect balance with other hormones.

Optimal levels are not high levels, though. Rather, they are the levels at which the body functions optimally. You don't want exceedingly high doses of hormones. When you give the body too much of a hormone, you get into trouble. For example, what do you think would happen if a woman gave herself exceedingly high doses of testosterone over a period of time? She would develop certain male traits! She might grow a few whiskers on her chin and upper lip, see her hair get thinner, become aggressive, gain a lot of muscle mass, think about sex a lot, and maybe even develop a larger clitoris. So, it is very important to find the right dosage and form of each bioidentical hormone you take.

Hormones need at least a week or two to start resolving your symptoms and it may take up to three months to find an optimal balance. Do not take it upon yourself to double your dosages early in treatment simply because you haven't felt any relief yet.

PREPARE FOR TREATMENT

The initial consultation with your doctor will include stacks of paperwork for you to fill out. The medical history form and symptom chart are the foundation of good communication between you and your health provider, so take time and thought in filling out these forms, as they will influence your therapy plan. Typically, progressive health providers will want to run comprehensive blood tests to see the status of your health and wellness. This is because symptoms can masquerade as hormonal, but may, in fact, be due to something entirely different (chronic infection, inflammation, neurotransmitter imbalances, or nutritional deficiencies). In fact, you should have all the following tests performed at the start of bioidentical hormone replacement therapy and every six months to a year thereafter.

- **Complete Blood Count (CBC).** Assesses numbers of red blood cells (RBC), white blood cells (WBC), hemoglobin, hematocrit, and the size of cells to help diagnose infection, anemia, and a number of other conditions.

- **Comprehensive Diagnostic Stool Analysis.** Tests the balance of normal bacteria and the presence of parasites or yeast overgrowth in the digestive tract, and evaluates digestion and absorption.

- **Comprehensive Metabolic Profile (CMP).** Includes electrolytes, sugar, protein, and kidney and liver tests to gauge organ function and overall health.

- **Delayed Food Sensitivity Test.** Involves maintaining a food diary and documenting your reactions.

- **Heavy Metal Test.** Tests levels of mercury, lead, cadmium, arsenic, aluminum, and other metals.

- **Hemoglobin A1c (HgA1c) Test.** Provides an average of the last few months of blood sugar levels.

- **Hormone Panel.** Evaluates hormone levels.

- **Immune Markers Test.** Looks at the cluster of differentiation 3 (CD3), CD4, CD8, CD19, complement component 3 (C3), lymphocytes, natural killer cells (NK), B cells, mature T cells, T-helper cells, T-supressor cells, antibodies (for example, IgG and IgE) detected against self (which give rise to autoimmune diseases), and antibodies detected against chronic infections (Epstein Barr, Cytomegalovirus, Human Herpes type 6, Lyme Disease, among others).

- **Inflammatory Markers Test.** Evaluates C reactive protein (C-RP), tumor necrosis factor alpha (TNF-alpha), interleukins, interferon gamma (IFN-gamma), homocysteine, fibrinogen, erythrocyte sedimentation rate (ESR), ratio of omega-3 to omega-6 fats (namely the ratio of arachadonic acid to eicosapentaenoic acid), uric acid, ferritin, plasma viscosity (PV), rheumatoid factor, creatine kinase, and antinuclear antibodies (ANA).

- **Iodine Test.** Checks levels of this mineral required for normal thyroid function.

- **Lipid Profile (including particles).** Gauges levels of lipoprotein a, apo lipoprotein A1 and B, remnant lipoprotein (RLP), dense LDL III and IV, VLDL, HDL and HDL 2b, triglycerides, and total cholesterol.

- **Neurotransmitter Profile.** Verifies levels of epinephrine, norepinephrine, dopamine, serotonin, glycine, taurine, GABA, glutamate, phenylethylamine, and histamine.

- **Nutrient Deficiency Test.** Evaluates gastrointestinal function, cellular energy production, nutritional deficits, protein adequacy, metabolic impairments, fatty acid levels, toxic metal exposure, and antioxidant reserves.

In addition, it is smart to get a physical exam that includes a blood pressure measurement, pulse reading, and bone density scan (called DEXA or DXA). Gynecological and breast exams, including a mammogram (or a Halo or thermogram) and a cervical Pap smear, are also recommended. Repeat these diagnostics yearly so you and your doctor can continue to weigh the risks versus the benefits of BHRT.

Testing Hormone Levels

As mentioned earlier, a hormone panel should be performed before you begin BHRT. There are three ways in which your hormone levels may be evaluated: by testing the blood, saliva, or urine. All three methods can provide useful clinical information about hormonal deficiencies and imbalances. Hormonal testing is a major component of attaining hormonal balance and should be discussed with your doctor to determine which type is best for you.

Blood Serum

Blood tests are the most common way to measure hormone levels. This may be because most health professionals are familiar with blood tests, and also because most insurance companies cover blood tests when a physician orders them for diagnostic purposes. Blood serum testing should be done between 7 and 8 AM after fasting for twelve hours in order to obtain accurate measurements of cortisol, insulin, and glucose. As there is no information determining the optimal amounts of estriol, thyroid antibodies, TPO, and SHBG, the normal ranges are used. Finally, while a blood test can be used to measure cortisol levels, a salivary test is generally thought to be a more accurate way to evaluate this hormone.

Saliva

Saliva testing is a popular alternative to blood testing. Proponents of this method say testing saliva better measures how well the tissues have taken up available hormones. Hormones floating around in the blood serum are bound to proteins and, therefore, unusable. As a result, serum levels may not be accurate, and may be out of sync with symptoms. Interestingly, free hormones (not bound to proteins) can enter the salivary glands. As a result, saliva gives a clearer picture of tissue uptake of free steroidal hormones, and may be a more accurate estimate of the quantity of free hormones reaching tissues. Also, while blood testing of hormones gives a snapshot of hormone levels at the time of the test, saliva testing reflects levels over several days. Saliva testing is also more comfortable (no needles), convenient, private (you can test from home), and often cheaper than blood testing (and is sometimes covered by insurance).

For accurate results, test multiple times throughout a day (for example, between 6 and 8 AM, 11 AM and 1 PM, 4 and 7 PM, and 9 and 11 PM), especially when testing the cortisol circadian rhythm. The most accurate results, in fact, are obtained by testing multiple days of the month. In addition, cortisol is best measured by a four-point salivary test. A DHEA level should also be drawn to calculate the optimal ratio of the two hormones. Take the sum of all four cortisol samples and divide it by the average DHEA level. The ratio should be about 5 to 1. If the ratio is higher, say 10 to 1, then you are producing too much cortisol.

Oral contraceptives or oral hormones may not be accurately reflected on this type of test. Your estrogen and progesterone may still appear low even if you are on oral hormones. If you are on bioidentical hormone replacement and want to test your levels via saliva, stop taking your supplements twelve to twenty-four hours before testing, otherwise the levels will appear elevated. While saliva is great for testing cortisol, estrogen, progesterone, and testosterone, it is not a suitable method for testing non-steroidal hormones such as insulin, thyroid hormones, or human growth hormone.

There is some skepticism over the accuracy of saliva testing (particularly for progesterone), but there is also well-documented research supporting this method of obtaining hormone levels. Talk to your health care provider about acquiring a saliva test kit.

Urine

In complex cases, I often encourage my patients to obtain their hormone counts via a urine test. This is the most accurate mode of hormone testing, but is also the most expensive and the most inconvenient—it involves collecting urine for twenty-four hours. It is my favorite test because it can provide information on the person's biochemistry as well as hormone levels. Biochemistry is important because it can guide your clinician in choosing one therapy over another.

For example, a urine test can show if you are converting the estrogen you naturally make (or take in) into harmful metabolites such as 16-alpha-OH estrone and 4-OH estrone. Specifically, it can tell you the ratio of benign estrogen metabolite 2-OH estrogen to dangerous estrogen metabolite 16-alpha-OH estrone. If it is greater than 2 to 1, your estrogen metabolism is good and you have a lower risk of breast cancer, lupus, and obesity. If the ratio is lower, DIM, the supplement that helps shift estrogen metabolism in the right direction, may be recommended, along with flaxseed, soy, omega-3 fatty acids, and exercise. If the ratio is too high, it can lead to bone loss, so a retest should be done in six months.

Additionally, after menopause, some women lack interest in sex even after taking testosterone. In such cases, a urine test that measures levels of bioavailable hormones and displays how well enzymes are working to metabolize these hormones can be helpful. If the test shows that bioavailable testosterone is low despite supplementation, the cause is likely an enzyme called aromatase, which can become overactive and cause testosterone to be converted into estrogen. This problem can easily be confirmed by a urine test, at which point your physician may suggest treating it with supplements such as flaxseed, grapeseed, and vitamin C, and by quitting smoking. Your pharmacist can also reformulate your testosterone prescription to include chrysin, a polyphenol that helps inhibit aromatase. In some cases a physician may recommend drugs that inhibit this enzyme, such as anastrozole, ketoconazole, or metformin.

Reference Ranges

In regard to diagnostic tests, results are compared to a reference range of what is considered normal. The normal range for hormone tests is not straightforward, though. It does not compare your readings with the vibrant hormone levels of a twenty-three-year-old woman. Instead, it compares them with those of other menopausal (or perimenopausal) women, who are all experiencing the natural drop in hormones that occurs with aging and stress. Obviously you will appear normal relative to that group of people, because they all have low levels. Women can have "normal" lab values for hormones but still experience menopausal symptoms because these values are not necessarily optimal levels. (Tell the younger ladies in your life who have no health issues or hormonal imbalances to get their hormone levels tested. This will be a valuable reference for them to consult when they experience perimenopause and menopause.)

Optimal blood serum reference ranges for each hormone have been determined, and they correspond to those normally found in healthy women between the ages of twenty-one and twenty-five. Increasing your hormone levels to these optimal ranges often eliminates deficiency symptoms, and may prevent the diseases commonly associated with aging. Optimal estrogen and progesterone levels in menopausal women, however, should be lower than those hormone readings in women of reproductive age, otherwise menstrual cycles would restart. It is my philosophy to give the lowest dosages of hormones to relieve menopausal symptoms and revive vitality, not to restore fertility.

The following table details the hormone levels that should be checked before the start of any hormone replacement program.

Each hormone has a standard reference range recognized by all medical professionals (which may vary slightly from lab to lab) and an optimal range recognized by progressive clinicians.

HORMONE REFERENCE RANGES		
Hormone	Standard Range	Optimal Range
Cortisol (Morning reading)	4.3–22.4 mcg/dL	10–14 mcg/dL
DHEA-S	42–290 mcg/dL	150–250 mcg/dL
Estradiol (E2)	less than 54 pg/mL	50–100 pg/mL
Estriol (E3)	less than 80 pg/mL	less than 80 pg/mL
Estrogen, Total	70–900 mcg/dL	61–437 mcg/dL
Estrone (E1)	12–41 pg/mL	20–95 pg/mL
Glucose, Fasting	65–99 mg/dL	70–85 mg/dL
Growth Hormone Marker (Somatomedin-C or IGF-1)	71–290 ng/mL	200–300 ng/mL
Insulin, Fasting	6–27 uIU/mL	less than 5 uIU/mL
Leptin	4–25 ng/mL	4–10 ng/mL
Pregnenolone	10–230 ng/dL	100–170 ng/dL
Progesterone	0–0.7 ng/mL postmenopause, 0.2–28 premenopause	5–20 ng/mL, 2–4 ng/mL if on transdermal progesterone.
Sex Hormone-Binding Globulin (SHBG)	18–114 nmol/L	18–114 nmol/L
Testosterone, Bioavailable (Free and weakly bound)	1.6–19.1 ng/dL	5–20 ng/dL
Testosterone, Free	0–2.2 pg/mL	1.2–6.8 pg/mL
Testosterone, Total	14–76 ng/dL	50–70 ng/dL
Thyroid, Active (Free T$_3$)	2.6–4.8 mcIU/mL	3.5–4.2 mcIU/mL
Thyroid, Inactive (Free T$_4$)	4.5–12 mcg/dL	8.25–12 mcg/dL

Thyroid, Reverse (Reverse T$_3$)	14.9–26.1 ng/dL	less than 25 ng/dL
Thyroid Antibodies	less than 20 IU/mL	less than 20 IU/mL
Thyroid Peroxidase Antibodies (TPO)	less than 35 IU/mL	less than 35 IU/mL
Thyroid-Stimulating Hormone (TSH)	0.35–5.50 mIU/mL	0.5–1.8 mIU/mL
Vitamin D, 25(OH)	20–100 ng/mL	60–100 ng/mL

If your hormone levels fall within the standard range, it is likely you do not have a debilitating hormone-related disease and your doctor will say that you are healthy. If your hormone levels fall outside the optimal range, you may not have a clinical disease, but you also may not function as well. You may complain of symptoms and have a decreased quality of life.

Standard Versus Optimal Saliva Cortisol Ranges

As noted earlier, cortisol is one hormone that may be better measured by a saliva test rather than a blood test. In addition, at least four salivary samples taken in the same day will be required to diagnose a cortisol imbalance. The following table lists the standard and optimal cortisol ranges according to the time of day this hormone is tested.

SALIVA CORTISOL RANGES		
Time of Day	**Standard Range**	**Optimal Range**
6–8 AM	1–8 ng/mL	3–6 ng/mL
11 AM–1 PM	0.2–3.5 ng/mL	0.5–2.5 ng/mL
4–7 PM	0.15–2.25 ng/mL	0.25–1.25 ng/mL
9–11 PM	0.1–1 ng/mL	0.15–0.5 ng/mL

Guidelines for Testing

If you are still having periods, test on day 20 or 21 of your cycle to measure peak progesterone levels. If you are no longer experiencing periods, you may take the test on any day of the month. If your cycles are extremely irregular and you can't pinpoint a day, you also may test any day of the month. If you are currently on some form of hormone therapy, you will need to stop it before testing. (Double check your testing instructions, as guidelines may vary.)

Some clinicians will even require daily four-point salivary cortisol tests over the course of one month to accurately understand your adrenal status.

Hormone Ratios

Even if you have optimal or normal levels of hormones, the ratio or balance of hormones can be off. Your progesterone-to-estrodiol ratio should be between 200 and 300 to 1, and your total testosterone-to-estrodiol ratio should be between 2 and 5 to 1. Be careful to watch your units! Have your health provider calculate them for you. This practice will provide a math tool that tells you if your hormones are out of balance. (Keep in mind that your symptoms will also reveal any hormonal imbalances.)

The Importance of Testing Hormone Levels

Some physicians may not be keen to test your hormone levels, and may say there is no scientific basis for such analysis. To be fair, hormone testing alone cannot paint the complete picture of your health. Your body requires not only the proper level of a hormone, but also the nutrients to activate that hormone, and a receptor that can receive that hormone's message. Your own specific hormonal balance can be best understood by considering both your symptoms and your hormone levels.

Most lab results of women in menopause show little to no estrogen, progesterone, or testosterone being produced. Commonly, perimenopausal estrogen levels are erratic on a daily basis, whereas progesterone is typically low throughout a given cycle. While there is truth in these statements, I find that taking a patient's medical history, symptom reports, and hormone levels before and during treatment yields superior management of her condition. This is because hormone laboratory values provide clinical goals against which results can be measured. Therefore, I always recommend that providers obtain hormone levels and symptom assessments before treatment and every six months to one year thereafter.

Hormone testing is a great tool your doctor can use to bring your hormones into balance. Of course, your symptoms will probably speak for themselves, but sometimes a hormone panel will reveal things that your symptoms do not and can guide your therapy accordingly. Retesting and follow-ups with your provider will promote the safety and effectiveness of your personal hormone plan.

SEX HORMONE REPLACEMENT

The following are dosage guidelines for estrogen, progesterone, and testosterone replacements for women going through perimenopause or menopause. Other details are outlined for those

Test Before Your Office Visit

Before you meet with a hormone specialist, you should arrange for your hormones to be tested. It is most helpful to know both your symptoms and lab results during a consultation so that the physician can effectively recommend the best regimen for your needs and goals. While each mode of testing has its virtues, your hormone clinician will be able to obtain valuable information from any type. I often recommend patients choose the cheapest testing method or one that is covered by insurance. (Call your insurance company to find out which one is covered).

with a high breast cancer risk. Typical dosage ranges are listed as a reference, but individualized hormone regimens designed by a physician may deviate from these limits, of course.

Estrogen

When estrogen is at optimal levels and in balance with other hormones, it produces many benefits in the body. When there is an excess or shortage of estrogen, uncomfortable symptoms and even debilitating health conditions can occur. As you know, hormone replacement therapy is used to help restore hormonal balance. Given the numerous adverse reactions linked to non-bioidentical hormone drugs like Premarin, however, I recommend instead that people take exact replicas of the same substances they have made naturally throughout their lives. This is what bioidentical hormone replacement therapy means. I also suggest that these hormones be put back at their right levels and in harmony with each other. BHRT users will feel better, age more gracefully, and, in my opinion, be safer than individuals who use hormones that are not identical to those produced by the human body.

The question is: When estrogen is supplemented, what is the proper balance of the different types of this hormone? The body makes the three estrogens in a particular proportion, producing 80 percent estriol (E3), 10 percent estradiol (E2), and 10 percent estrone (E1). In light of this fact, some physicians prescribe an estrogen supplement called triest, which reflects these amounts. The truth is, however, that estrone replacement is likely unnecessary. Women still make enough of this form of estrogen after menopause. Given the risk of creating more of estrone's harmful immediate metabolites (16-alpha-OH estrone and 4-OH estrone), I prefer the estrogen supplement known as biest (also called diest). It contains 80 percent estriol and 20 percent estradiol. Moreover, I have recently begun to recommend biest at the ratio of 50 percent estriol to 50 percent estradiol, since estriol can inhibit estradiol's action, making it seem like the estrogen supplement is not working. This concentration is also preferred if a patient wishes to avoid weight gain. Be mindful of your estradiol dose, though. Remember, it causes cell growth in breast and uterine tissues. (Many studies suggest the total estradiol daily dose should be less than 0.1 mg for transdermal patch preparations.) For breast cancer survivors, if any estrogen is to be given, estriol alone should be given vaginally, while estradiol and estrone should be avoided.

Never take estrogen by mouth. An oral preparation goes from the gut straight to the liver, promoting the buildup of xenoestrogen metabolites. If you are currently taking an oral estrogen, taper off of the dosage and then trade it in for a topical or sublingual preparation. These formulations bypass the liver and go to the tissues first, minimizing the production of carcinogenic metabolites.

If you take or used to take an oral estrogen preparation, take a course of milk thistle for three to four weeks as well as an ongoing treatment of DIM to help clean your liver and push estrogenic metabolism toward benign metabolites. You can do both treatments at the same time. The liver can be cleansed further with added dietary supplements and lifestyle changes. The following guidelines may help detoxify your liver:

- Eat a diet that includes flaxseed and soy-rich foods.

- Exercise for thirty to ninety minutes most days of the week.

- Take 1 g of omega-3 fatty acids four times a day.

- Take 150 to 300 mg of DIM per day.

- Take 200 mg of milk thistle three times daily for three to four weeks.

Another option for estrogen replacement is estrogen pellets. These compressed hormone pellets, which are the size of a grain of rice, are placed underneath the skin. As the release of hormone is constant, this may be the best option for those who have trouble remembering to take medications daily, as well as those who have severe symptoms that last both day and night. The pellets last a few months. Their downsides are their cost and the fact that you are stuck with a particular dosage once they are inserted. If the dosage chosen at the time of insertion is not optimal, you will feel uncomfortable and have to make another trip to the doctor for an adjustment.

As estrogen levels decline during menopause, vaginal tissue atrophies. The vagina tends to feel extremely dry, the walls thin, and sex can be extremely painful. Vaginal estriol cream or suppositories plump up the vaginal tissue and get the juices flowing again. Initially, 1 mg of estriol can be inserted into the vagina each night at bedtime for about two weeks. As symptoms resolve, it may be used two to three times a week. If you are sexually active, it is best to engage in intercourse before inserting estriol, so as not to pass along the hormones to your partner.

Breast Cancer Survivors

It is impossible to extend an open invitation to all breast cancer survivors or those at high risk of breast cancer to use estrogen in the treatment of severe symptoms of menopause. I do, however, have some tips for those who have weighed the increased risk of breast cancer against menopausal symptom management and still want to try hormonal therapy. The only option is vaginal estriol, and it should be accompanied by vaginal progesterone and vaginal testosterone preparations. But consider this only after a full physical and gynecological workup by a physician, and after lab tests have confirmed the need for supplementation. Of all estrogens and routes available, low-dosage vaginal estriol accompanied by progesterone and testosterone is the only hormone replacement option for select high-risk patients. Still, risks versus benefits must be weighed.

Progesterone

If you are supplementing estrogen, don't be afraid to add progesterone, even if you don't have a uterus. Estrogen was made to work together with progesterone, and progesterone was made to balance the effects of estrogen. Giving one without the other may throw your hormones off balance, promoting estrogen dominance.

Usually perimenopausal conditions require progesterone supplementation without the addition of estrogen. This is because the body has enough estrogen during this stage (especially if there is a buildup of xenoestrogens). Progesterone is needed to prevent the symptoms of estrogen dominance. But if you take progesterone and are still cycling, you will need to vary the dosage throughout the month to maintain a regular cycle. Progesterone might be taken on days 14 to 25 or 12 to 26 of your cycle to imitate your body's natural monthly progesterone flux. There is no harm in giving progesterone daily, but periods may be irregular. Some cycling patients have severe symptoms of estrogen dominance throughout the month and may prefer to supplement progesterone on days 1 to 25 or 5 to 26.

If one of your severe symptoms is insomnia, and you are already taking topical or sublingual progesterone at bedtime, try switching to an oral preparation of progesterone (never take oral estrogen, as you know). Progesterone will go straight to the liver and will break down into compounds that help you sleep. The only oral progesterone dosages commercially available are 100 and 200 mg, which are suspended in peanut oil. The dosage of topical preparations is about a quarter the dosage of oral formulations. You might need a specific amount for your situation, which may be compounded at a compounding pharmacy.

Natural Phytoestrogens Versus Bioidentical Estrogens

Phytoestrogens are naturally occurring estrogen-like substances found in many herbs (such as black cohosh) and soy foods. These products are weaker than and different in structure from human estrogen. They can still help alleviate mild menopausal symptoms as well as estrogen dominance and are available at health food stores as supplements, but they will not transform into human-identical estrogen in the body.

I usually advise patients to avoid taking progesterone in the morning or during the day. This is because progesterone can help you get to sleep (even the topical and sublingual preparations). If you have severe anxiety during the day, however, splitting your dose into a twice-daily regimen may help you relax, improve your mood, and keep progesterone levels constant.

When you meet with your hormone specialist for BHRT, it is important to discuss any history of progestogen supplementation. Whether you are taking Provera for menopausal symptoms or using a typical birth control pill for pregnancy prevention, it should be disclosed to the doctor you see for hormone management. This information, combined with your symptom list and health status, will influence your prescriber as to the best bioidentical hormone regimen for your system.

Testosterone

All tissues in the body have testosterone receptors. As such, testosterone can send messages to your hair, skin, bone, heart, brain, eyes, fat, muscle, and so on. For example, testosterone may tell the skin to produce more sebum, or the vagina to produce more secretions and dilate blood vessels during sex, or fat cells to shrink and muscle mass to increase. Testosterone benefits the body when its level is optimal and in balance with other hormones. If there is an excess or shortage, uncomfortable symptoms and health problems may occur. If a woman's testosterone level exceeds its optimal amount, she may experience male-typical conditions, such as facial hair and male-pattern baldness. If her testosterone is too low, her sex drive could be non-existent.

There is currently no testosterone replacement product commercially available for use by women. Products such as Androgel contain too much testosterone for a woman. While a commercial bioidentical testosterone product with a lower concentration should be on the market one day soon, for now, compounded testosterone products are a woman's only option for prescription testosterone replacement. They are often topical or sublingual preparations.

Although testosterone may be prescribed to enhance energy and increase metabolism, there is also a complicated but effective way to use this hormone to raise libido. This may be done by applying your topical testosterone dose to your inner arm or thigh one morning and then applying it directly to your clitoris or inner labia the next day instead. Using more than 0.5 mL of cream on this area can be messy, so make sure the concentration is formulated to account for this fact. Also take note that topical testosterone has about a four-hour lag time in promoting sexual desire, so plan accordingly. You can repeat this schedule (i.e., apply your usual dose on most days of the week and then apply it directly to the clitoris in place of your method two to three times a week). If you find that the positive libido effect begins to wear off after a while, your receptors are probably saturated. In this event, stop taking the testosterone completely for about two weeks. You may then resume testosterone use as before. This practice revives the sensitivity of hormone-tolerant receptors.

If you need to replace testosterone but are afraid of or are starting to exhibit male physical characteristics, it might be a good idea to try substances that reduce testosterone such as spironolactone (100 mg daily), saw palmetto (160 mg of standardized extract daily), finasteride (5 mg daily), or metformin (500 mg three times daily). Ask your physician first, however, if one of these medications might be right for you, as they can have other effects on the body and are conventionally used to treat other conditions.

When you meet with a hormone specialist for BHRT, be sure to discuss your history of testosterone supplementation. In particular, it will be helpful for the specialist to know if you have ever used testosterone replacement therapy (either bioidentical or not) and why you stopped taking it, if applicable. This information, combined with your symptom list and health status, will influence your prescriber as to the best testosterone dosage for your body.

Finally, it is important to note that testosterone can make insulin resistance worse. On the other hand, testosterone helps burn fat, builds muscle, and increases metabolism, which can prevent insulin resistance. When taking testosterone, monitor your blood sugar level, triglycerides, weight, waistline, and blood pressure.

Switching from Synthetic to Bioidentical Hormones

If you have been on artificial estrogen or progestin prescriptions for the relief of your symptoms, there are a few steps to take when switching to bioidentical hormones. You can stop the oral progestin and switch to bioidentical progesterone, either oral or topical, right away. Meanwhile, the switch to bioidentical estrogen should be done in stages. Transition to oral triest first, and then to oral biest (50 percent estriol and 50 percent estradiol), and then to topical biest (50 percent estriol and 50 percent estradiol). During this period, I generally recommend supplementing with 150 mg DIM daily and 220 mg milk thistle three times daily for three to four weeks.

Women already using transdermal bioidentical estradiol patches may feel symptoms of estrogen dominance. This is because estradiol patches tend to raise serum estradiol levels much more than creams. Making the switch to topical compounded biest cream may be a better option for estrogen dominant women on estradiol patches. While some research suggests that 1.5 mg estradiol gel is equivalent to the 0.05 mg estradiol patch, saliva testing shows that the 1.5 mg topical gel gets more estrogen to tissues than the 0.05 mg transdermal patch. Therefore, I hardly ever recommend switching to 1.5 mg of topically applied estradiol, as it is just too potent. Rather, I would recommend starting with biest (50 percent estriol and 50 percent estradiol) at a dosage of 1 mg, which contains only 0.5 mg of estradiol. Reassess your condition in one week. I would expect a call from a patient within a few days if the new dosage were too low. (Hot flashes and night sweats would have returned by that time.)

An Example of Switching

As an example of how to make the transition from non-bioidentical to bioidentical hormone replacements, let's look at a patient who takes 0.625 mg of Premarin and 5 mg of Provera per day but wishes to switch to bioidentical hormone replacements. Provera can be stopped immediately and replaced with bioidentical progesterone. An equivalent dosage would be either 200 mg of oral progesterone or 50 mg of topical progesterone.

A Premarin dosage of 0.625 mg is about the same amount as 2.5 of oral triest (80 percent estriol, 10 percent estradiol, and 10 percent estrone) or 1 mg of biest (50 percent estriol and 50 percent estradiol), and switching to one of these choices must be done in the following stages:

- Discontinue Premarin.

- Take 2.5 mg of oral triest for two to four weeks.

- Switch to 1 mg of oral biest (50 percent estriol and 50 percent estradiol) for two to four weeks.

- Switch to 0.5 mg of topical biest (50 percent estriol and 50 percent estradiol) for two to four weeks.

- Finally, taper to 0.2 mg of topical biest (50 percent estriol and 50 percent estradiol), which may not be easy or ever attainable, since Premarin's potency may have made your body accustomed to a very high level of estrogen supplementation.

Separate Containers

When you begin hormone replacement therapy, ask that each of your hormones be dispensed in a separate container. This allows individual adjustment of hormone dosages as you find the right balance. After you and your doctor have found a stable dosage of estrogen and progesterone, hormones may be combined for convenience. (This option is often cheaper too.) Keep your testosterone prescription separate from the other hormones, however, if you want to use it to increase libido.

Cleanse your system, as previously mentioned, starting on the day bioidentical estrogens are introduced. Begin with 150 mg of DIM daily and 220 mg of milk thistle three times daily for four weeks. DIM may be continued for another few months or indefinitely to ensure that xenoestrogens are properly eliminated.

Dosage Chart

The following hormone dosage ranges are based on my own clinical experience as well as the work of consultant pharmacists Jim Paoletti and Monica Kaul and breast cancer surgeon Rebecca L. Glaser. Clinical trials have used dosages within these ranges.

SEX HORMONE DOSAGE CHART		
Hormone	**Dosage**	**Considerations**
Biest, Topical (50 percent estriol and 50 percent estradiol)	Start with 0.5–1 mg per day until specified by your physician. Continue with maintenance dosage of 0.1–0.5 mg per day.	**For Patients in Perimenopause:** If progesterone alone doesn't control symptoms, give cyclically on days 1–25. May not need as much as menopausal women. Start with low dosage (0.05–0.25 mg) and adjust slowly. **For Patients in Menopause:** May use continuously or include a 3–5-day holiday per month. **For Patients with Breast Cancer Risk:** Use vaginal estriol only. Do not use estradiol. Insert 0.25 mg daily for two weeks, and two to three times per week thereafter.
Biest, Topical (80 percent estriol and 20 percent estradiol)	Start with 1.25–2.5 mg per day until specified by your physician. Continue with maintenance dosage of 0.25–1.25 mg per day.	**For Patients in Perimenopause:** If progesterone alone doesn't control symptoms, give cyclically on days 1–25. May not need as much as menopausal women. Start with low dosage (0.125–0.625 mg) and adjust slowly. **For Patients in Menopause:** May use continuously or include a 3–5-day holiday per month. **For Patients with Breast Cancer Risk:** Use vaginal estriol only. Do not use estradiol. Insert 0.25 mg daily for two weeks, and two to three times per week thereafter.

Hormone	Dosage	Considerations
Estriol, Vaginal	Start with 1 mg at bedtime for two weeks, and then use two to three times per week as needed for vaginal atrophy.	**For Patients in Perimenopause:** May not need as much as menopausal women. **For Patients in Menopause:** May use in addition to topical biest preparations in cases of severe dryness or atrophy. **For Patients with Breast Cancer Risk:** Use lower dosages of 0.25 mg daily.
Progesterone, Oral (Sustained-release)	25–400 mg per day.	**For Patients in Perimenopause:** Take on days 14–25 or every day with a 3–5-day holiday per month. This is the best formulation for insomnia. **For Patients in Menopause:** May use continuously or include a 3–5-day holiday per month. May not need as much as perimenopausal women. **For Patients with Breast Cancer Risk:** Take 50–200 mg daily. May cause yeast overgrowth, which the supplement *S. boulardii* (1 billion organisms per capsule) may help prevent.
Progesterone, Topical	10–200 mg per day.	**For Patients in Perimenopause:** Take on days 14–25 or every day with a 3–5-day holiday per month. **For Patients in Menopause:** May use continuously or include a 3–5-day holiday per month. May not need as much as perimenopausal women. **For Patients with Breast Cancer Risk:** Use 25–50 mg (topical or vaginal) daily for two weeks, and two to three times per week thereafter.
Testosterone, Topical	0.25–4 mg each morning.	**For Patients in Perimenopause:** May not need as much as menopausal women. **For Patients in Menopause:** May use. **For Patients with Breast Cancer Risk:** Use 0.25mg (topical or vaginal) every morning for two weeks, and two to three times per week thereafter.

All daily doses may be divided into a twice-daily regimen. For example, 50 mg of progesterone daily may be taken as two doses of 25 mg, one in the morning and one in the evening. This method is helpful when a patient has anxiety during the day. Finally, the textbook *Basic and Clinical Endocrinology* suggests a daily topical estradiol dose between 0.05 and 0.1 mg, but the amounts in clinical practice have been higher. Therefore, it is best to discuss your individual regimen with your provider.

METABOLIC HORMONE REPLACEMENT

Diet and exercise are excellent natural ways to increase your metabolism and build a beautiful, healthy body. Unfortunately, as women approach menopause, the hormones in charge of metabolism begin to decrease. Without the help of your hormones, you may work twice as hard and eat half as much as before but achieve only minimal weight loss.

The main hormones involved in energy and metabolism are testosterone, DHEA, cortisol, and thyroid hormones T_3 and T_4. Additionally, insulin must be kept in check by following a healthful diet, and serotonin levels must be sufficient to keep cravings away. Balancing these metabolic hormones should lead to true weight-loss results. If they are not at optimal levels, your waistline may keep growing and your energy may continue to lessen.

Benefits of Balanced Metabolic Hormones

Before you consider using hormone replacement therapy to balance your metabolic hormones, it is important to remember the numerous benefits of these hormones. Once you recognize how vital metabolic hormones are to your health, you will have any easier time following your BHRT plan. Your hormone regimen will seem worth it as you look forward to the fantastic results you can achieve with BHRT.

- **Cortisol.** Increases blood pressure and heart rate, decreases digestion, preserves energy stores, mobilizes blood glucose and amino acids to use on demand, decreases amino acid uptake by muscles, acts as a diuretic, promotes fat storage as a means of self-preservation, and performs many other functions in response to stress.

- **DHEA.** Decreases the formation of fat, promotes weight loss and lean muscle mass, and increases insulin sensitivity.

- **Human Growth Hormone.** Promotes cellular rejuvenation, tissue repair, wound healing, bone density and strength, brain function, and hair and nail strength.

- **Insulin.** Regulates blood sugar levels in the body and enables cells to convert glucose into energy. Without insulin, the body would not be able to harness glucose for energy, as seen in people with diabetes.

- **Melatonin.** Promotes deep sleep and bone growth, acts as a powerful antioxidant, improves mood, boosts immunity, increases tolerance to stress, inhibits premature aging, and stimulates human growth hormone production.

- **Pregnenolone.** Increases resistance to stress, improves energy and sleep quality, reduces pain and inflammation, and elevates mood.

- **Serotonin.** Calms mood, promotes satiety, and helps manage food cravings.

- **Testosterone.** Maintains and promotes muscle mass and strength, decreases body fat, increases exercise tolerance, protects against cardiovascular disease, improves cholesterol, and enhances a sense of well-being.

- **Thyroid Hormones.** Controls body temperature, energy production, and the metabolic function and growth of every cell.

Unfortunately, the aging process and lifestyle choices can cause these hormones to fall out of balance. Whether there is a hormone deficiency or excess, an imbalance will cause a number of reactions in the body. The following table matches each hormone with the metabolically related symptoms that can occur when its level is not optimal.

	SYMPTOMS OF METABOLIC IMBALANCE	
Hormone	**Symptoms Due to Deficiency**	**Symptoms Due to Excess**
Cortisol	Anorexia, chronic fatigue, fibromyalgia (muscle and joint aches), hypoglycemia (low blood sugar), diabetes, intolerance to high-potassium foods in the morning, more effort required to do everyday tasks, swollen ankles in the morning, and cravings for foods high in fat, salt, or caffeine.	Abdominal weight gain, insulin resistance, difficulty losing weight, fatigue, heart disease, high cholesterol, and water retention.
DHEA	Raised blood pressure, elevated cholesterol, diabetes, decreased energy, decreased muscle mass, obesity, and poor fat metabolism.	Acne, increased hair growth, oily skin and hair, and skin rash.
Human Growth Hormone	Elevated serum lipid concentrations, increased fat mass (especially around waist), decreased bone density, lowered exercise tolerance, decreased immune function, reduced muscle mass, reduced vigor and optimism, and a higher risk of death from heart disease.	Carpal tunnel syndrome, headaches, muscle and joint pain, poor glucose tolerance, and swelling.
Testosterone	Abdominal weight gain, difficulty losing weight, raised cholesterol, lack of energy, poor exercise tolerance, reduced strength and endurance, poor muscle definition and mass, and decreased tendon and joint health.	Increased muscle mass, insomnia and excessive energy, and elevated levels of aggression and assertiveness.
Thyroid Hormones	Elevated cholesterol, excessive fatigue, heart palpitations, muscle and joint pain, slowed heart rate, unexplained weight gain, and water retention.	Fatigue, feeling nervous or anxious, osteoporosis, racing heart, shakiness, trouble sleeping, and warmer body temperature.

Considering all the health troubles that follow a metabolic imbalance, and knowing the positive effects that accompany the restoration of metabolic hormones to optimal levels, it is clear that BHRT may be of use to individuals who are affected by this problem. A closer look at these is warranted.

DHEA

DHEA helps optimize metabolism, energy, and immunity. While this hormone tends to decline with age, be sure to test your DHEA level before you supplement. If you are not deficient but take a supplement anyway, the excess DHEA may be converted into other hormones and create an imbalance. Both symptoms and confirmed levels of low DHEA suggest you may be a candidate for supplementation. Although you can buy DHEA supplements over the counter, be wary of their quality. Since the FDA does not heavily regulate dietary supplements, the actual content of DHEA may be different than what is stated on the package. In addition, the over-the-counter DHEA supplements are typically not formulated as sustained-release preparations, so you have to keep taking them throughout the day to keep your levels up. Moreover, typical DHEA preparations are available in 25-mg and 50-mg oral dosages, which are appropriate for use by men, but women usually need only 5 or 10 mg. If your doctor has prescribed DHEA, the best option is pharmaceutical-grade sustained-release DHEA (DHEA-SR) from a compounding pharmacy. A compounding pharmacy can also make other forms of supplemental DHEA, such as sublingual drops or lozenges, or topical creams or gels to meet your unique needs.

If you would like to use DHEA primarily for weight loss, 7-keto-DHEA may be a better choice than regular DHEA. Unlike regular DHEA, this form of DHEA does not convert into other hormones, though it can produce similar benefits in the body. Because it does not convert into testosterone, it may be used by women who have facial hair or acne without fear of worsening those conditions.

Human Growth Hormone

If you have been diagnosed with human growth hormone deficiency, replacement therapy will help you retain lean muscle and lose fat. Since human growth hormone is a peptide hormone, it is injected under the skin. Don't be scammed by vendors offering sublingual sprays or oral tablets of hGH. Often a daily injection of 0.2 mg is a reasonable starting dosage of human growth hormone. Some products express their dosages in IU, so it should be noted that 1 mg is equivalent to 3 IU. A prudent clinician will recheck the hormone levels at three weeks and then decide if an adjustment should be made. The typical maintenance dosage for women is 0.35 mg daily and 0.6 to 2 mg daily for men. Be ready to pay a lot of money for this hormone. It may cost more than a thousand dollars per month. (Omnitrope and Saizen tend to be cheaper than Genotropin.)

While growth hormone supplementation can be a therapeutic option for those with a deficiency, studies have linked many adverse effects to high levels of hGH, including swelling, increased blood pressure, insulin resistance, and joint and muscle pain (namely carpel tunnel syndrome). The trouble may be the high dosages subjects were given in these studies. A smaller daily dosing regimen that closely mimics natural hGH secretion should lead to better outcomes and fewer adverse events.

Nevertheless, sometimes it seems that the risks of hGH supplementation outweigh the benefits. This is why you may see the FDA cracking down hard on doctors who prescribe this particular hormone as if there were no medical risk associated with it. The FDA does, however, recognize human growth hormone deficiency as a medical condition and permits the supplementation of hGH by prescription. If your growth hormone levels are low and you have the symptoms of low hGH, you may qualify for growth hormone supplementation. To screen for growth hormone deficiency, you will need to obtain a serum somatomedin-C (also called IGF-1) level. Doctors screen for this related substance because human growth hormone has a half-life of only fourteen

---

Hormone Holidays

Taking a break from hormone treatment can keep your body sensitive to these supplements. Too often, after a couple of months of daily use, hormones don't work as well as they once did. During your hormone regimen, take Sundays off, or take a three-day block off each month. Hormone holidays are recommended for DHEA, testosterone, pregnenolone, and melatonin. Thyroid and cortisol hormones should be taken daily. Human growth hormone requires a three-week holiday after every five-month treatment period.

---

minutes in the body, whereas IGF-1 stays around for twenty-one hours. IGF-1 should optimally be between 290 and 400 ng/mL.

Some providers encourage their patients to take three-week breaks from treatment about every five months. This hormone holiday helps keep your pituitary working properly. If hGH supplementation is not right for you, you can also make certain lifestyle changes to increase your growth hormone production naturally.

Testosterone

Testosterone replacement therapy is quite a powerful tool for boosting energy levels, increasing lean body mass, and encouraging the loss of fat. Typically people feel its metabolic effects within a couple of weeks of starting treatment. If you are afraid that testosterone replacement will produce male characteristics like facial hair, ask your physician whether it can be taken along with other supplements that may decrease these reactions, such as saw palmetto.

Avoid oral testosterone preparations; they won't absorb well and will get chewed up in the liver. Injectable forms will release very high levels of this hormone during the first few days and slowly fall thereafter, causing a yo-yo effect. Testosterone pellets (inserted under your skin by a physician) can be an option if you are on a stable dosage. The pellets last between three and five months and are the best choice if you have trouble remembering to take your testosterone as prescribed.

Personally, I prefer creams for testosterone replacement. When properly applied to the inner arm or inner thigh, the cream absorbs well and releases hormone slowly into the blood stream. Levels will remain therapeutic during the day and fall by evening so you will be able to sleep well. Vaginal creams and suppositories are especially effective at enhancing libido, but may not reach the rest of the body.

Thyroid Hormones

Hypothyroidism is usually treated with a T_4 supplement known as levothyroxine (Levothroid, Levoxyl, or Synthroid). While T_4 is the inactive thyroid hormone, most people respond well to this therapy. As the body ages, however, the enzyme responsible for converting T_4 into the active T_3 is produced less or is not as active. In this case, supplements cannot address the signs and symptoms of low thyroid hormones. If you find that you are low in free T_3, or that your hypothyroid symptoms are not relieved by a T_4 supplement, consider taking a T_3 supplement, which may better address the underlying issue.

Long-acting T_3 preparations compounded by a pharmacy will have fewer side effects than immediate-release T_3 products, such as Cytomel. This is because immediate-release preparations cause a quick spike of thyroid hormone in the blood, which can temporarily feel like hyperthyroidism. In addition, immediate-release T_3 must be taken two or three times daily, which can be difficult to remember. I have, however, recommended long-acting thyroid preparations over immediate-release versions to certain patients who suffer from digestive issues (specifically poor absorption caused by irritable bowel syndrome or leaky gut syndrome). This type of patient isn't able to absorb the hormone through the stomach lining very well and therefore doesn't respond successfully to therapy. If you think you may have a gut absorption issue, it may be best to stick with an immediate-release thyroid preparation.

Compounding pharmacies can make thyroid prescriptions in any combination of T_4 and T_3 required. If you meet with a hormone specialist who can analyze your symptoms, lab tests, and previous thyroid regimen history, you should be able to receive a treatment plan that will include a specific combination dose of T_4 and T_3 hormones. Sometimes your needs will match a commercially available product that contains both hormones, such as Armour thyroid or Nature-Throid. These products are pig thyroid gland extracts and consist of four parts T_4 and one part T_3 per tablet. The benefit of taking gland extracts is that they also contain essential minerals such as selenium, zinc, magnesium, and iodine, which the thyroid requires to function properly. They also contain thyroid metabolites T_2 and T_1, which may or may not possess hormonal activity. You may find you need a compounded version, though, due to an aversion to porcine products or because you require a unique ratio of T_4 to T_3. The human body actually makes T_4 and T_3 in a 3.3-to-1 ratio, not the 4-to-1 ratio found in porcine thyroid extract.

People who can't convert T_4 to T_3 well will find they benefit from a 2-to-1 or 1-to-1 ratio of T_4 to T_3, or from just T_3 by itself. In these cases, a compounded thyroid medication is best and the compounding pharmacy can include minerals if your doctor asks them to do so.

Excess Thyroid Hormones

Thyroid supplementation can give you more energy and increase your metabolism, but if your dosage is too high for your body, you may experience symptoms of hyperthyroidism. Your heart may seem to beat too fast, and you may feel hot, sweat more, or even feel anxious. When starting a new thyroid regimen, make sure your physician is available to recheck your levels in three months or as needed. This will ensure that you don't receive a dosage of thyroid supplements that is too high. Sometimes, however, hyperthyroidism is a natural phenomenon. Either way, its signs should not be ignored.

The following are the typical symptoms a woman experiences when her thyroid levels are high. If you have more than half of these conditions, it is likely that your thyroid is out of balance.

- Diarrhea
- Dizziness
- Fatigue
- Feeling nervous or anxious
- Heart palpitations
- Hot flashes and sweating
- Increased appetite
- Increased body temperature
- Itching and hives

- Light or missed periods
- Muscle weakness
- Osteoporosis
- Paralysis
- Shakiness
- Thinning hair
- Trouble sleeping
- Vision changes
- Weight loss

If you switch compounding pharmacies, your levels might also fluctuate slightly due to the difference between pharmacy formulations. The differences should be miniscule, but it is a good idea to inform your physician of the potential for fluctuation.

Dosage Chart

Your doctor will typically start you at low metabolic hormone dosages and adjust slowly up or down to reach optimal levels. Adjustments to thyroid hormone supplements can be made after one week, but most are adjusted every two to four weeks. There is no agreed upon protocol for hormone replacement therapy at this time, but I personally have found that many patients do well within the following ranges.

This information is in no way meant to supersede your doctor's orders and is based on my own clinical case studies. Some cases will fall outside the ranges listed, but the majority of

Vitamin and Mineral Supplements for Low Thyroid Levels

A low thyroid level can bring about nutritional deficiencies. It reduces production of hydrochloric acid in the stomach, and therefore fewer amino acids are absorbed by the body. Some progressive physicians load their patients with intravenous therapy when beginning thyroid treatment. These nutrients are required by the enzyme that converts T_4 into T_3.

The following substances are generally administered via IV to patients on hormone replacement therapy:

- Calcium gluconate: 100–300 mg
- Chromium piccolinate: 200 mcg
- Magnesium: 2,500 mg
- Selenium: 40–200 mcg
- Tailored amino acid therapy (especially tyrosine)
- Vitamin B Complex 100: 4,000 mg
- Vitamin B_{12}: 4,000 mcg
- Vitamin B_6: 100 mg
- Vitamin C: 10,000 mg
- Zinc sulfate: 1–5 mg

Note that iron and vitamins A (10,000–25,000 IU), D_3 (10,000 IU), and E (1,000 IU) are also required but are usually given orally on a daily basis, not via IV.

patients will achieve optimal hormone levels and alleviate their symptoms within these limits. Always talk to a health professional before beginning a hormone regimen to optimize your energy and metabolism. Typical dosage ranges are listed for your reference, but your particular hormone regimen as designed by your physician may deviate from these numbers.

METABOLIC HORMONE DOSAGE CHART		
Hormone	**Starting/Upper Limit Dosages**	**Considerations**
DHEA, Topical	1 mg–10 mg per day	Used in place of oral DHEA when patient has excess estrogen. Use starting dosage to manage mild symptoms. Adjust to achieve desired effect. Recheck level in six months.
DHEA S, Oral	5 mg–15 mg per day (some doctors go up to 50 mg per day)	Use starting dosage to achieve desired effect. Recheck level in six months.
7-Keto-DHEA, Oral	25–200 mg per day	Used in place of DHEA when patient has oily skin, facial hair, or excess weight. Use starting dosage to manage mild symptoms. Adjust to achieve desired effect.
Human Growth Hormone, Injectable	0.2–0.6 mg per day	The usual maintenance dosage is 0.35 mg per day six days a week. Take hormone holidays. Norditropin can be stored at room temperature for three weeks.
T_3 S, Oral	5–40 mcg per day	Use when only T_3 is low. Use non-SR if there is poor stomach absorption. Use starting dosage when there are no symptoms. When symptoms exist, start with 5 mcg in morning and at noon. Adjust to achieve desired effect. Recheck level in three months.
T_4 and T_3 SR, Oral (80 percent T_4 and 20 percent T_3)	18–144 mcg of T_4 per day, 4.5–36 mcg of of T_3 per day	Use when both T_4 and T_3 are low. If more T_3 is needed, use a formulation of 75 percent T_4 and 25 percent T_3. Use non-SR if there is poor stomach absorption. Use starting dosage when there are no symptoms. When symptoms exist, start with 36 mcg of T_4 and 9 mcg of T_3. Adjust to achieve desired effect. Recheck level in three months. May add 2 mg of zinc picolinate, 10 mg of magnesium glycinate, 0.075 mg of potassium iodide, and 0.05mg of selenium per capsule.
Testosterone, Topical	0.5–6 mg per day	The usual dosage is less than 4 mg per day. Best taken in the morning. Symptoms of excess androgen may be decreased by such substances as saw palmetto, metformin, finasteride, and spironolactone.

HORMONE REPLACEMENTS FOR STRESS AND BURNOUT

Of course, the most important treatment for stress and burnout involves learning how to handle and reduce stress in the first place. While this is the most vital part of therapy for stress, hormone supplements can also help if you are already faced with high cortisol levels or adrenal exhaustion.

Adrenal Concentrate

Adrenal concentrate, which is extracted from the adrenal glands of cows, can supplement cortisol levels. This product may be purchased over the counter and is an excellent therapy for adrenal fatigue. Oral formulations are recommended at a starting dosage of 80 mg per day. This amount may be raised to the upper limit of 220 mg if necessary.

Melatonin

The body produces less than 0.3 mg of melatonin each day. Levels can drop with age, causing problems with sleep. Without proper sleep, your body will not be able to heal and regenerate itself properly. In addition, you will not be able to make other hormones optimally. There is currently no standard dosage schedule for melatonin supplementation, and each person responds differently to treatment. Typically, over-the-counter products offer dosages between 0.3 and 5 mg. Oral or sublingual formulations are recommended and should be taken about thirty minutes prior to bedtime. Supplementation may cause morning drowsiness. If your starting dosage of melatonin makes you very drowsy quickly, begin with an even lower amount. It is also a good idea to have your melatonin level tested before beginning supplementation.

Due to melatonin's pivotal role in sleep, supplementation may help you fall asleep faster, stay asleep longer, be more alert during the day, and prevent or ease jet lag. Typically, a dosage of 3 to

Melatonin and Breast Cancer

Low melatonin levels may be linked to an increase in breast cancer risk. Women with breast cancer often have lower levels of melatonin than those without the disease. In addition, low levels of
melatonin stimulate the growth of certain types of breast cancer
cells, while adding melatonin to these cells inhibits their growth.
Melatonin may also enhance the effects of certain chemotherapy
drugs used in the treatment of breast cancer. If you have (or have
had) breast cancer, talk to your doctor to see if melatonin supplementation is right for you.

6 mg of melatonin taken thirty to sixty minutes before bedtime
should help you achieve these results. If melatonin supplementation causes you to be drowsy throughout the day, try a lower
dosage. Keep in mind that high amounts of melatonin may cause
anxiety, vivid dreams, and irritability. In addition, if you plan to
take melatonin for sleep, you may only need a few weeks of treatment to get your sleep cycle back.

By increasing serotonin production, melatonin may also help
treat depression, anxiety, and seasonal affective disorder (SAD, a
mild depression associated with lack of sunlight in the fall and
winter). The combination of melatonin supplements and certain
antidepressant medications carries potential risks, however, so
melatonin should be used only under the direct supervision of
your physician. The melatonin dosage to treat depression is usually 0.125 mg taken twice daily at 4 PM and 8 PM.

Due to melatonin's potential side effects and the risk of this
hormone interacting with other medications, you should consult
with your doctor before starting any melatonin regimen.

Pregnenolone

Your doctor may suggest pregnenolone supplementation to treat
adrenal dysfunction. Of course, levels must be tested first to con-

firm the need to supplement. It's also important to check cortisol levels at this time, since a need for increased cortisol production robs your body of available pregnenolone. While there is no standard dosage for pregnenolone supplementation, I usually recommend taking 5–25 mg once to twice a day. Low dosages of 1 mg per day may help with sleep quality, while high-dosage injections of up to 500 mg per day may help with rheumatoid arthritis pain. Pregnenolone is available over the counter as a pill, but it can also be taken under the tongue. Additionally, it may be compounded with other hormones or supplements. Pregnenolone's possible but rare side effects include headaches, irritability, insomnia, heart palpitations, and acne.

Cortisol

Cortisol is a last resort in the treatment of adrenal fatigue. It should be used only after all lifestyle modifications and other nourishing supplements have been tried for one to three months with little success. Low dosages of bioidentical cortisol treatment given for a short period of time can allow the adrenals to take a rest and become healthy again. The typical dosage can range from as little as 1.25 mg once in the morning with breakfast to 15 mg twice daily with meals. The amount should be adjusted by your doctor every month or so based on your symptoms. Treatment can last between three months and two years. Long-term treatment, however, is discouraged due to possible immune suppression. The key is to keep in close contact with your doctor. Monthly or quarterly check-ups are often warranted to achieve positive results.

Cortisol is bioidentical and may be compounded as an oral sustained-release preparation at a compounding pharmacy. There are also commercially available products, namely Cortef. Cortef tablets are immediate-acting oral preparations and are available in 5-mg, 10-mg, and 20-mg dosages. Some patients prefer the instant energy surge offered by Cortef over the sustained-release cortisol compounds, but either option is a reasonable choice.

Thyroid and Cortisol

If you don't treat your cortisol imbalance, you may shift your thyroid hormones out of balance or cause an established thyroid problem to become much worse. For example, if you treat a hypothyroid condition before dealing with adrenal fatigue, your cortisol level will drop even more! Thyroid hormones speed up the breakdown of cortisol in the body. Thus, it is important to treat both adrenal insufficiency and hypothyroidism simultaneously; or, even better, heal the adrenals first and then use thyroid supplementation. Conversely, if you treat a hypothyroid issue during a high-cortisol period, the thyroid supplement won't work effectively. This is because excess cortisol can cause protein carriers to bind to thyroid hormones. This decreases the available free thyroid hormones, which may encourage the hypothyroid symptoms you're trying to address. In this case, getting the cortisol under control first will not only help your adrenals, but will also free up your own thyroid hormones, and you may not even need thyroid supplementation.

CONCLUSION

The basic treatment principles and dosage ranges outlined in this chapter can be extremely useful for those who are taking or considering taking bioidentical hormones to manage the symptoms of perimenopause or menopause. Of course, finding the right balance between estrogen, progesterone, and testosterone can be tricky. It usually takes time and patience to regain optimal hormone levels. With the right knowledge and a compassionate health care provider, however, your body can be brought back into balance. Combined with some of the lifestyle changes and dietary choices mentioned on the following pages, you can feel healthy and vibrant again.

4

Alternatives to Hormone Replacement Therapy

Hormone replacement therapy is not for everyone. There are some women who should probably consider other treatments for the symptoms associated with menopause and other age-related conditions. For example, a woman who has breast cancer (especially estrogen-receptor-positive breast cancer), unexplained genital bleeding, liver disease, or is prone to blood clots or pregnant should definitely consider alternatives to BHRT. If bioidentical hormone replacement therapy is not right for your situation, explore the lifestyle changes, dietary options, nutritional supplements, and possibly even prescription drugs that may help you feel healthy again. (While I rarely recommend the commercially available prescription drugs mentioned in this section, the most common ones are listed here for your information.) There are many alternative treatments for issues such as menopause, insulin resistance, decreased metabolism, and stress. As always, though, speak with your health care provider to determine the best treatment for each of your symptoms or conditions.

NON-HORMONAL TREATMENTS FOR SYMPTOMS OF MENOPAUSE

While hormone therapy can make you feel better quickly, it is only one way to live well both during and after menopause. Taking a holistic approach to this stage of life is the key to feeling better. The most important choice you can make is to adopt a healthy lifestyle. If you smoke, quit the habit. Smoking decreases estrogen levels and makes the transition through menopause much harder. Other lifestyle changes include being physically active every day, eating a variety of fruits and vegetables, increasing your intake of lean protein (chicken, fish, beans, soy), limiting your alcohol consumption (if you drink regularly, try to cut back and switch to red wine), limiting saturated fat and cholesterol in your diet (most fat should be unsaturated—with the one exception being virgin coconut oil—and from plants, such as olive oil, or from fish such as salmon), decreasing the stress in your life, and maintaining a healthy weight.

While these general health tips can help restore your overall well-being, not all women experience the same number of symptoms to the same degree during menopause. You may be looking to focus on one or two of the conditions associated with this stage of life, and fortunately there are more specific alternative treatments for these problems.

Hot Flashes and Night Sweats

Hot flashes can have a debilitating effect on a woman's quality of life. For those who experience raging hot flashes constantly, a decrease in the severity and frequency of these attacks would most certainly be welcomed. But can it be done without the help of hormone therapy? Absolutely, it can. A few simple lifestyle changes can help alleviate or prevent a hot flash. If these do not help, supplements may be considered.

Lifestyle Changes

Wear light fabrics such as linen or cotton, and avoid synthetic fibers like polyester. If you live in a cool climate, layer your clothing. Avoid spicy foods, caffeine, and foods that promote heartburn. Sleep in a cool room. Engage in stress-reducing activities such as yoga or meditation, deep breathing, exercising and stretching regularly, lying down during breaks at work, going to sleep early, minimizing interactions with the stress-inducing individuals in your life, finding laughter each day, and confiding in friends and family when you're faced with difficult situations.

Phytoestrogens and Herbs

Phytoestrogens are estrogen-like substances derived from plants. Since they are weaker than human-identical estrogens, they may relieve mild hot flashes, but aren't typically the answer for severe hot flashes. They can also be useful in those with estrogen dominance because they occupy the estrogen receptor in place of the more potent human estrogen. They help decrease lipids and provide cardiovascular protection. They can be consumed through foods or supplements. Sources include foods such as soy and yams, and herbs such as black cohosh, dong quai, and valerian root. A diet rich in soy will include tofu, tempeh, soymilk, and soy nuts.

PHYTOESTROGEN AND HERB DOSAGE CHART		
Supplement	**Dosage**	**Instructions**
Black Cohosh	40–80 mg	Take one pill twice a day. Preparation must be standardized to contain 1 mg of triterpene 27-deoxyactein per 20 mg.
Dong Quai	0.75–30 mg	Typical dosage is 4.5 mg once a day.
Evening Primrose Oil	500 mg	Take once a day.
Phytoestrogens	40–80 mg	Consume this amount daily. Whole foods rich in soy are a better choice than phytoestrogen supplements.
Valerian Root	2–3 g	Typically taken one to three times a day. Valerian has been studied in connection with only four to six weeks of use. It should not be taken for any longer without the supervision of a health care provider.

Unfortunately, there is no solid evidence that phytoestrogens actually relieve hot flashes. In addition, the risks of the more concentrated forms of soy, such as pills and powders, are not known. Certain phytoestrogens may worsen estrogen-receptor-positive cancers and should be discussed with your doctor before starting. An alternative option to phytoestrogens, evening prim-rose oil not only helps relieve hot flashes but also lessens PMS symptoms and breast tenderness.

If you decide to try any of these options, consult the previous table for dosages and discuss your regimen with your health care provider.

Vaginal Dryness

The decrease in estrogen during menopause causes thinning of the vaginal wall and an increase in vaginal pH. This leads to painful intercourse and frequent yeast or bacterial infections of the vagina and urinary tract. Having sex regularly can increase blood flow to the vagina and help maintain vaginal health. There are also some other ways to improve the situation.

Probiotics

Probiotics can help restore the pH balance. These are the good bacteria that can help stop pathogenic bacteria and yeast from thriving in the vagina. A compounding pharmacy can prepare vaginal suppositories containing healthy probiotic strains, such as *Lactobacillus acidophilus*. Oral probiotics can help as well. A personal favorite is one that contains *Saccharomyces boulardii*. While *S. boulardii* is yeast itself, it acts like a policeman for other yeasts and removes them from your intestinal bacterial garden. The typical regimen is to take one capsule orally once to twice daily.

Vaginal Lubricants

Over-the-counter water-based personal lubricants may help with dryness, but occasionally a large amount is required for relief, which can be messy. The lubricants do not relieve itching and do not address the thinning of the wall. A vaginal moisturizer such as KY Long-Lasting Vaginal Moisturizer may be a better choice, since it lasts longer and replenishes the water content of the vagina. Additionally, if a more natural approach is desired, compounding pharmacies can create vitamin E vaginal suppositories or creams.

Vaginal Spasms, Bladder Spasms, and Pelvic Pain

Many women who have given birth will complain of chronic vaginal spasms or bladder spasms that may be accompanied by pain. This condition can be quite uncomfortable and concerning. Some menopausal women who have never been pregnant or given birth can also experience this phenomenon, although it can happen at a much younger age as well.

Medications

Treatments for these issues include non-hormonal local (vaginal) anti-spasm medications such as baclofen and cyclobenzaprine, neuropathic (nerve) pain medications such as gabapentin, lidocaine, and amitriptyline, and anti-anxiety medications such as diazepam. The best results usually come from a combination product, of which there are two popular examples. The first is a vaginal cream that consists of 2.5 percent baclofen, 6 percent gabapentin, and 2.5 percent amitriptyline. The second is a suppository that contains 10 mg of cyclobenzaprine, 5 mg of diazepam, and 62.5 mg of lidocaine. Both products are inserted vaginally (or sometimes rectally) up to four times a day (but usually starting one time daily at bedtime). While I don't like using pharmaceutical drugs, in cases such as these, where the cause of the issue is most likely anatomical changes or nerve damage to the area, they may be the best option. Taking these types of medication by mouth can cause serious side effects, including dizziness and drowsiness, which is why I recommend drugs that are applied close to the problem area.

Libido and Sexual Dysfunction

More than 40 percent of American women have trouble achieving orgasm. This number includes young ladies not yet experiencing perimenopause or menopause, but also counts perimenopausal or menopausal women with diabetes, heart disease, or hardened arteries, who have a tough time achieving orgasm due to a lack of blood flow to the clitoris. Testosterone replacement can sometimes correct the issue by increasing vaginal lubrication, heightening stimulation, and increasing blood flow to the genitals, but there are non-hormonal options that can work wonders as well.

Scream Cream

There are a handful of non-hormonal therapies that effectively address both female and male sexual dysfunction. Many of these options work by increasing blood flow to the genitalia or by priming the area for heightened sensation. As a compounding pharmacist, I have prepared the most popular compounds that have helped women perk up their sex lives. The most famous in the compounding pharmacist's world is called "Scream Cream." Each gram of cream contains 30 mg of aminophylline, 2.5 mg of isosorbide-dinitrate, 0.5 mg of ergoloid mesylate, and 50 mg of pentoxifylline. Sometimes 60 mg of the amino acid L-arginine is added as well. Those with genital herpes, however, should not apply L-arginine because it promotes the growth of the virus. Your pharmacist will use a hypoallergenic base that allows for fast absorption but local action (which means fewer side effects). To use the cream effectively, apply 0.25 to 0.5 g to the clitoris five to thirty minutes before sex. Its effect can last for up to two hours.

Other Drugs

Sildenafil, the generic of Viagra, is also a popular topical compound with female patients who wish to enhance blood flow to the clitoris. Other drugs known to help are nifedipine, papaverine, and phentolamine.

Excess Estrogen

Some women naturally make ample amounts of estrogen due to an overactive enzyme called aromatase that converts testosterone to estrogen. Typically, these women have normal amounts of progesterone. As a result, they can have estrogen dominance even before perimenopause begins. The danger is that too much estrogen can cause cancer. So, if you are one of the many women who naturally produce loads of estrogen yet have perfectly normal progesterone levels, you may need to decrease your natural estrogen production. Progesterone is an anti-estrogen, and you are certainly welcome to supplement it to match the excess of estrogen, the trouble is that you can end up feeling quite hormonal with high levels of both sister hormones. The other way to approach the situation is to take a medication that inhibits the conversion of testosterone into estrogen.

Medications

One drug that inhibits the conversion of testosterone into estrogen is called anastrozole. If you were to search this on the internet, you would find it is used as breast cancer chemotherapy. While it may sound scary, this drug is only going to dampen the effects of your overactive estrogen production and can correct the imbalance. Taking a very low dosage can be just the trick you need to get your estrogen levels back on track. Let your doctor determine which amount might suit your body. A dosage of between 0.025 and 0.5 mg should be fine. Take one capsule orally three times a week or once daily. You shouldn't experience any side effects at that dosage level, but if your physician gives you a dosage that is too high for your body, you will experience menopausal symptoms due to low estrogen levels. Check your estrogen levels after four to six weeks or at the onset of low estrogen symptoms.

Mood Swings

Mood swings may be the most disturbing symptom of your experiences with perimenopause and menopause. One minute you're happy, the next sad, and later on angry and tearful. Many people around you will be insensitive to menopausal mood swings and will cut you no slack when you express your internal emotional struggle. But what can you do if you don't qualify for or are weary of taking hormones to level out these roller-coaster moods? Typically, your doctor will promote the use of anti-depressants, but you can also take charge by reducing your stress levels, increasing sleep, avoiding toxins, maximizing nutrition, and balancing your neurotransmitters.

Lifestyle Changes

It is very important that you get seven or eight hours of restful sleep each night. Also, be physically active. Exercise will not only help you sleep but can also raise your level of endorphins, which make you calm and happy. Caffeine, nicotine, and alcohol must be limited or eliminated, as they can alter your mood. Additionally, reduce your stress levels. If your primary symptom is anxiety, cognitive behavioral therapies can help a lot. For example, make a list of situations that make you feel anxious, put them in order with the easiest last, and then work your way up the list, purposefully exposing yourself to the stimuli that make you increasingly anxious. If you are feeling angry, you can focus on the situations or people that make you angry and then confront them.

Supplements

Neurotransmitters are chemicals that act as messengers for the brain. They might better be called "brain hormones." Neurotransmitters are made using amino acids and nutrients as their starting materials. They regulate processes such as sleep, energy, digestion, metabolism, interest in sex, pain perception, hormone regulation, and mood. The most widely studied neurotransmitters are dopamine, epinephrine (adrenaline), gamma-aminobutyric acid (GABA), glutamate, glutamine, histamine, norepinephrine, and serotonin. Nearly 80 percent of people have some level of neurotransmitter imbalance, which may be a root cause of depression, anxiety, insomnia, attention deficit disorder, fibromyalgia, migraines, obesity, PMS, irritable bowel syndrome, and many other disorders. This imbalance can be caused by a genetic predisposition, chronic stress, drugs (both illicit and prescription), toxic chemical exposure (heavy metals, pesticides), or poor nutrition.

Tailored amino acid replacement therapy and proper nutrition can often normalize a neurotransmitter imbalance. Both neurotransmitter testing and amino acid testing are necessary to create such a therapy. Your health care provider will be able to assess your levels and devise a regimen to fix the imbalance. Nutritional deficiencies have been implicated in this issue, so pinpointing the nutrients you lack and correcting the problem could also promote your overall health.

Both depression and anxiety are often associated with a lack of serotonin. Usually, my first choice for boosting natural serotonin production is a supplement of the amino acids L-tryptophan (500 mg once to three times a day) and 5-hydroxytryptophan (200 mg one to two times a day). In addition, vitamin B_6 (pyridoxine), vitamin B_3 (niacin), and glutathione (the body's major detoxifying compound) are needed to convert tryptophan into serotonin. Iron, vitamin B_3, and vitamin B_7 (biotin) are required to regulate serotonin levels. The amino acid taurine may also help lift depression. Your body needs zinc, magnesium, vitamins A and B_6, and cysteine to maintain proper taurine levels.

Other natural treatments for depression and anxiety include tyrosine, phenylalanine, L-dopa, yohimbine, guarana, rhodiola, and a high-protein diet. In dealing with anxiety specifically, the neurotransmitter GABA and the amino acid glutamate can be calming. Glycine, B vitamins, branched-chain amino acids, and a complex carbohydrate diet can also help calm a restless mood. Vitamin B_8 (inositol) can improve both depression and anxiety. Once your provider has checked your personal neurotransmitter and nutritional imbalances, optimal dosages of these substances may be determined. Many progressive and integrative physicians' offices are equipped to provide intravenous vitamin therapy tailored to your particular needs.

Antidepressants and Anti-Anxiety Drugs

If anxiety is a major problem, SSRIs (selective serotonin re-uptake inhibitors) are viable options. SSRIs keep serotonin from being re-absorbed by serotonin-producing neurons. If you find you are still anxious after taking an SSRI for a few weeks, the benzodiazepine class of medications (Ativan, Valium) might be helpful, but these drugs tend to make you drowsy, and you can become dependent on them. In general, these drugs do not address the root cause of your problems; they only address symptoms. In addition, chronic consumption of these drugs may deplete your natural reserves of neurotransmitters. What's worse, high doses of SSRIs may be needed to maintain the desired effect. Also, if the serotonin-producing cell needs to make more reserves constantly, serotonin resistance can occur. It's no wonder that this class of drugs is accompanied by dangerous side effects (including suicidal tendencies in young people). For this reason, I promote treating the cause and not the symptom. Therefore, I suggest testing for and treating neurotransmitter and nutritional imbalances before opting for prescription drugs.

Dilantin

Dilantin is a medication that is known for treating seizures. It is not as recognized for treating depression and anxiety, but is quite effective in managing these conditions. To understand why this medication is effective, picture the brain made up of nerves, which act like wires, carrying electric current from one place to another. When you are anxious, depressed, or can't sleep, this electricity surges and causes static, and low dosages of dilantin can calm these surges down. Dilantin can also help with migraines, concentration or memory problems, hyperacivity, and substance withdrawal. The common dosage of dilantin is one 100-mg capsule taken orally twice a day.

Insomnia

Sleep is central to a healthy and vibrant life. The best way to repair the body and adjust to stress is to engage in deep sleep for eight hours or more (starting before midnight). Stress and menopause are two conditions that tend to disrupt sleep patterns, which impacts your overall health and contributes to weight gain.

Sleep Habits

Changing your sleep habits, perhaps with the support of a sleep specialist, is the single most effective therapy for insomnia, no matter what the cause. Good sleep habits can increase the quality and quantity of your sleep, without the risk of dependency on sedative hypnotic medicines. First, set a regular time to go to bed as well as a regular time to wake up. Engage in consistent moderate exercise, preferably early in the day, avoiding strenuous activity late in the day (exercise increases your metabolism and energizes you). Evening exercise, however, is better than no exercise, so don't use insomnia as an excuse to get out of exercising. Avoid daytime naps whenever possible. Avoid consuming caffeine in large amounts or after noon. Minimize alcohol consumption at all times. While alcohol can initially make you drowsy, it can also cause midnight awakening or fragmented sleep. Don't eat heavy or spicy meals late in the evening; this can disrupt both your digestion and your sleep. A warm shower or bath immediately before going to bed can be soothing and relaxing. A glass of warm milk or a cup of yogurt before bed may make you drowsy, as these contain melatonin, serotonin, and tryptophan.

Make the bedroom as quiet and comfortable as possible, with no clocks in sight, and reserve it only for sleep and sexual activity (although some find it very restful to watch TV in bed). To get into the mood to fall asleep, try soothing music, audio hypnosis, dim lighting, or a relaxing book. If you are trying to sleep but are not asleep within thirty minutes, move to another room and do an easy activity or task until you become drowsy. If you can't stay asleep because you are worrying about the upcoming day's events, get up and make a list of the tasks ahead so that you won't forget them. This will help your brain turn off.

Supplements

After changes in sleep habits, alternative medicines are the second line of the treatment for insomnia. Kava kava is a Fijian remedy for insomnia, anxiety, and seizures. Kava kavalactones, which are the extracted active ingredient in kava kava, may be supplemented at a dosage of 100 to 200 mg a day, while 1 to 3 g of kava kava root may be taken per day. This supplement is metabolized heavily by the liver and should not be taken with alcohol. As previously mentioned, L-tryptophan is an amino acid from which the body synthesizes serotonin. When serotonin is made, it improves the quality of sleep, lessens anxiety and depression, and helps you cope with stress. A dosage of 500 mg of L-tryptophan should be taken at bedtime and repeated one time that night if needed.

Magnesium is a mineral that becomes depleted after many nights of sleep deprivation. This mineral is responsible for hundreds of bodily functions. Low magnesium levels have also been linked to restless leg syndrome and anxiety. Daily supplements of 1,000 mg of magnesium should help. Finally, valerian root has sedative and antidepressant properties and is well tolerated. Take one 600-mg pill of valerian root (the ethanolic extract) thirty to sixty minutes before bedtime.

Pharmaceutical Sleep Aids

As always, drugs should be your absolute last option in addressing health issues. Fix the cause of insomnia and you can avoid these drugs entirely. You may try over-the-counter sleep aids such as Benadryl or Unisom, but for a maximum of only seven days. Any longer and you will build tolerance, and they won't work as well anymore. They are also notorious for causing a morning "hangover," dry mouth, and constipation. Avoid the routine use of prescription sedative hypnotics such as Restoril, Ambien, Lunesta, and Sonata. While they work rapidly, tolerance develops quickly (as soon as three nights). If you use them regularly and want to stop taking them, be sure to taper off gradually to avoid rebound insomnia. Finally, trazodone, an approved treatment for depression, is often prescribed for the treatment of insomnia because it is a non-addictive option.

Memory and Concentration Problems

Difficulty with concentration and memory is one of the most common cognitive complaints of the menopausal woman. Foggy thinking can be frustrating and even affect job performance in severe cases. While estrogen activates neurotransmitters and dilates blood vessels in the brain, there are other non-hormonal ways of improving memory and concentration. These remedies are not found in a prescription pill, but rather through changing key lifestyle behaviors and seeking alternative medications. And don't forget to remove the cause (if known) of brain fog. Stress plays a role in memory. The more stressed you are, the harder it is to remember things. Another cause of memory loss is a high level of heavy metals, such as mercury, in the body. Chelation therapy and the avoiding of these metals will help improve your memory and cognition.

Lifestyle Changes

Getting enough restful sleep is important for maintaining mental acuity and memory. Sleep relaxes and rejuvenates the body and mind. Being physically active also gives your brain a workout, creating more neurotransmitters and endorphins. Cardiovascular exercises also clean plaque from your arteries, reducing your risk of stroke. Mental exercises and critical thinking may also be used to keep your brain sharp. Some studies even suggest that people who engage in regular critical thinking have a lower chance of developing Alzheimer's disease.

Supplements

If you have severely foggy thinking, memory lapses, or attention deficit disorder, consider having your nutritional status tested, including amino acid and vitamin levels. Excellent memory aids include 5-HTP, lipoic acid, omega-3 fish oil, acetyl-L-carnitine, and phosphatidyl serine. Regimens will vary from person to person.

In addition, gingko biloba is an herb that may enhance memory. The usual dosage of gingko biloba leaf extract is 600 mg per day. The extract should be standardized to 24 percent flavones and 6 percent terpene lactones. Furthermore, panax ginseng root extract promotes proper cognitive function at dosages of 100 to 400 mg per day. The extract should be standardized to 4 to 7 percent ginsenosides. Also worth exploring are food sensitivities. People who have difficulty concentrating may be constantly eating foods that their bodies cannot tolerate.

Osteoporosis

There is well-documented research that a lack of estrogen accelerates bone loss and the progression of osteoporosis. Women in menopause, having a lack of estrogen, are at higher risk of getting osteoporosis. If hormone replacement therapy has been excluded as a treatment option, there are other things you can do to prevent or address osteoporosis.

Lifestyle Changes

There are many simple ways to reduce your risk of osteoporosis. A sedentary lifestyle is a risk factor for osteoporosis, so keep moving. Do thirty minutes of weight-bearing exercise three times a week, which should maintain bone density. If you are past menopause, over sixty-five, or have a history of hip fractures, get a bone mineral density screening. A DEXA scan of the hip yields the most precise results. Reduce risk of falls by having annual eye, hearing, and nerve exams. Also, avoid medications that inhibit balance, such as sleep aids. Finally, don't smoke.

Supplements

Since 99 percent of your body's calcium supply is stored in bone, when blood levels of calcium are too low or your pH is too acidic, your body leeches calcium from the bone to try to temporarily correct the deficiency or restore pH balance. That's why getting enough dietary calcium and maintaining a healthy diet are essential ways to protect bone density. Foods rich in calcium include certain fish (salmon and sardines), leafy greens (spinach, Brussels sprouts, collard greens), tofu, beans, almonds, peas, dairy products (milk, yogurt, cottage cheese), and fortified juices. I discourage the consumption of dairy, however, since it is a strong source of inflammation. If you don't think you are getting enough calcium from your diet, you will have to take supplements. Calcium hydroxyapetite is a superior formulation, as it is the most absorbable form and contains the same ratio of calcium to phosphorus as human bone. You can take 500 mg three to four times a day. Be aware that calcium supplements tend to cause stomach upset, gas, and constipation. These side effects happen less frequently with calcium citrate preparations. Also, calcium can leech thyroid medications and iron supplements if taken at the same time, so be sure to take these substances at least an hour or two apart. Calcium supplements must always be balanced with magnesium. Typically the ratio is one part magnesium to two parts calcium. Therefore, a dosage of 500 mg of magnesium taken once to twice a day should be sufficient. Vitamin D helps increase the dietary absorption of calcium into the bone. Sources of vitamin D include fish (salmon, mackerel, tuna, sardines, and cod liver oil), fortified milk and cereal, eggs, beef, liver, and sun exposure. You may also take vitamin D supplements, but have your doctor check your level before deciding on a dosage.

Selective Estrogen Receptor Modulators (SERMs)

SERMs decrease bone loss by selectively stimulating the estrogen receptors of the bone without stimulating the receptors of the breast or uterus. This is a great treatment option for osteoporosis patients who are at high risk of breast or uterine cancer because the drug does not promote these cancers. Evista is usually taken as a 60-mg tablet once a day. Femarelle is taken twice a day in capsule form (322 mg of tofu extract, 108 mg of flax seed). The draw-backs are that this class of drugs (especially Evista) can sometimes worsen hot flashes and promote blood clotting.

Bisphosphonates

This class of drugs is traditionally considered a first-line treatment to stop the progression of bone loss. It has been shown to increase bone mineral density and prevent hip and vertebral fractures. (Calcium and vitamin D must also be supplemented if dietary intake is not sufficient.) Bisphosphonates work by preventing natural bone breakdown mechanisms. In other words, they encourage old bone to remain part of the skeletal structure. They do not, however, increase bone strength.

You must take the medication first thing in the morning (before any food or drink) and be able to sit or stand for the following thirty minutes to an hour. This type of drug can aggravate gastroesophageal reflux disease (GERD). Luckily, its half-life is very long, so you can get away with taking it once a week (Fosamax or Actonel), once a month (Boniva), or even once a year (Reclast). This medication must be administered by a health care professional.

Hypertension and Coronary Heart Disease

Coronary heart disease is a leading cause of death and loss of quality of life in women. The risk for hypertension and coronary heart disease increases after menopause. Certain factors such as increasing age, obesity, diabetes, smoking, and physical inactivity are correlated to this risk. Conventional medicine states that high cholesterol levels lead to clogged arteries and decreased blood flow, which is the perfect recipe for a heart attack or stroke. Typically, doctors prescribe a statin drug such as Lipitor or Crestor to lower cholesterol. I do not believe these cholesterol-lowering drugs will save everyone from heart disease. While they are good at lowering LDL and have anti-inflammatory effects, they come with many side effects, including muscle weakness, pain, and inflammation. Other possible side effects include liver dysfunction and the depletion of coenzyme Q_{10}.

Like high cholesterol, hypertension is also generally treated with pharmaceuticals. The most commonly prescribed classes of medications for high blood pressure are thiazide diuretics, ACE inhibitors, angiotensin II antagonists, beta-blockers, and calcium-channel blockers. Like cholesterol-lowering drugs, these medications can have side effects. Overall, I usually don't recommend taking them unless your doctor says they are absolutely necessary. Thankfully, there are other ways to prevent these dangerous conditions.

Lifestyle Changes

If you are overweight or obese, losing weight is the single most important lifestyle change you can make to reduce your risk of cardiovascular disease. Those who maintain an ideal body weight lower their risk of developing cardiovascular disease by 35 to 55 percent. The NIH has recommended a diet called Dietary Approaches to Stop Hypertension (DASH), which is rich in potassium and calcium, and low in sodium (only 1 teaspoon allowed per day). Total fat consumption should be limited to 25 to 35 percent of total daily calories, while saturated fat should be under 7 percent. You should eliminate trans fats entirely from your diet and increase your fiber intake to between 25 and 50 g per day (soluble fiber especially helps maintain blood sugar). Optimal glucose levels will prevent the many cardiovascular complications that come with diabetes. Thirty to ninety minutes of daily physical activity five to seven days a week is another important habit. Limit alcohol consumption to one to two drinks per week.

Monitoring your blood pressure at home may help you maintain these changes. Also, know the signs and symptoms of a heart attack (chest pain, shortness of breath, nausea, and light-headedness) or stroke (numbness on one side of body, trouble speaking or understanding, trouble seeing or walking, and severe headache) so that you may seek help immediately in the face of one of these conditions.

Chelation Therapy

Chelation therapy with EDTA disodium has been shown to help reverse hardened arteries. It acts by removing the calcium deposits along arteries, thus enhancing their flexibility. This therapy is considered experimental by traditional standards, but is being done at progressive physicians' offices every day. A typical regimen as recommended by the ACAM (American College for Advancement in Medicine) is to give 1 to 3 grams of EDTA intravenously over four hours. Your doctor may also add magnesium, B vitamins, and vitamin C. Therapies are repeated up to three times a week for about thirty treatments. At the end of your treatment course, your physician will reassess your cardiovascular condition. Care should be taken to not to decrease blood calcium levels too low.

Supplements

A natural approach to lowering blood pressure begins with diet, of course, but if you still need a bit of help, magnesium supplementation may be able to provide it. Taking 300 to 500 mg per day along with your daily supplement of 800 to 1,000 mg of calcium can be effective in lowering blood pressure in some cases. A more aggressive approach to decreasing blood pressure (as well as breaking up clogged arteries) may be magnesium sulfate intramuscular injections (given as 1 g once a week). In addition, intravenous phosphatidylcholine drips can help dissolve cholesterol plaques and renew cell membranes. Finally, coenzyme Q_{10} (100 to 300 mg a day), L-carnitine (1 to 3 g a day), and L-arginine (500 to 3,000 mg a day) may also reduce blood pressure.

Hair Loss

It's not just men who can lose their hair; women can, too. Of course, the pattern of hair loss is different in women. Typically, there is no receding hair line but rather a diffuse loss of hair on the entire top portion of a woman's head. Hair loss in women can be due to a number of reasons. The loss of estrogen production during menopause can be a major culprit. Those who naturally produce more androgenic hormones (testosterone, DHT) due to genetics or environment will complain of hair loss. Women with low thyroid hormone levels or those who are stressed out and thus have soaring cortisol levels may also live through a hair-loss nightmare. Aside from hormonal imbalances, nutritional imbalances can also be a cause of this problem.

Testosterone Conversion

A shampoo that contains pantothenic acid (vitamin B_5), biotin, and azelaic acid (which prevents the conversion of testosterone into DHT, a common cause of hair loss in men) can help prevent hair loss. Additionally, the topical medication minoxidil is known to inhibit the conversion of testosterone into DHT. It is available over the counter for both men and women. If the cause of hair loss is stress, there are natural ways to reduce this emotion. (These techniques are detailed on page 160.)

Skin Changes

Muscle under the skin tends to become smaller as we age, which makes the skin sag. In addition, hormonal imbalances such as high or low cortisol levels, estrogen dominance, and pregnancy can cause dark spots to occur. Conversely, light patches can happen if your thyroid hormone levels are too high or too low, if cortisol is too high or too low, or if sugar and insulin levels are consistently elevated.

Prescription Cosmeceuticals

One of my favorite pastimes at the pharmacy is preparing novel fruit-acid foaming face washes, potent wrinkle creams, acne gels, antioxidant serums, and post-laser masks. A favorite combination product that I use for dark spots contains hydroquinone (6 percent), hydrocortisone (1 percent), retinoic acid (0.1% percent), and kojic acid (3 percent). I also love a particular antioxidant wrinkle cream I make that contains ubiquinone (coenzyme Q_{10}), ascorbic acid (vitamin C), alpha lipoic acid, and DMAE in varying concentrations. The options are infinite for a custom beauty product prepared by a pharmacist. Your doctor can change the concentration of any active ingredient and concoct a unique cosmetic treatment just for you. If you are allergic to certain chemicals or would like a more natural base, your requests can be met.

Laser Treatment

A wide variety of laser treatments can promote collagen and elasticity, and remove wrinkles and sunspots. These procedures are the most expensive way to manage skin issues, but yield superior results.

Vitamin and Mineral Treatment for Overall Relief

Vitamins and minerals are essential to health. When they become depleted, the body cannot function as it should. There are particular vitamins and minerals that are vital to hormone production and balance, and supplementing with these substances can help bring overall relief to the symptoms that accompany menopause. The following list details these items and their common dosages:

- **Boron Aspartate or Citrate.** Boron is essential for estrogen and testosterone production, and it helps prevent calcium loss in bone. Dietary sources include dates, prunes, raisins, nuts, and honey. It may be supplemented at 1.5 to 3.5 mg a day.

- **Folic Acid.** Folic acid, also known as vitamin B_9, helps promote DNA repair, which is one way the body prevents cancer naturally. Supplement with 0.25 to 1 mg a day. Better yet, try folinic acid, the activated form of folic acid, at 800 mcg a day.

- **Vanadium.** The proper vanadium level is essential to maintaining the right progesterone level. Too much can create progesterone loss and not enough can create progesterone excess.

Take 13 to 26 mcg a day, or as needed, and have your vanadium level tested whenever possible.

- **Vitamin A.** This vitamin is essential to making hormones. Take 5,000 to 10,000 IU a day.

- **Vitamin C.** This vitamin is also needed to make hormones. The ester form of vitamin C is fat soluble and may be easier to absorb than other chemical forms. Take 500 to 1,000 mg a day.

- **Vitamin E.** Vitamin E is not only a powerful antioxidant, but can help relieve hot flashes. Studies have associated low vitamin E levels with decreased hormone production. Take 400 IU twice a day.

- **Zinc.** Zinc is required for estrogen receptors to function properly, is a cofactor in hormone synthesis, protects the breast from cancer, and promotes bone formation. Take 25 to 50 mg a day.

Unless they are suggested by your physician, you will not need iron supplements if you have stopped menstruating for more than a year. Those who are still menstruating or have heavy periods due to perimenopause may benefit from 325 mg (65 mg of elemental iron) of daily ferrous sulfate supplementation. Serious cases of ongoing menstrual bleeding, however, may require a higher amount to prevent anemia.

NON-HORMONAL TREATMENTS FOR INSULIN RESISTANCE

Glucose, a simple sugar, is a cell's main fuel source and is required for the body to function. Insulin, a hormone secreted by the pancreas, helps regulate blood sugar levels in the body. Insulin helps the cells take in glucose and convert it into usable energy. Without insulin, glucose levels would build up in the blood after a meal because the body would not be able to harness the glucose for energy.

Optimal levels of glucose in the blood, when measured after fasting, are between 70 and 85 mg/dL. When cells become resist-

Stem Cell Therapy

Right now your body holds the key to your health and wellness in a line of cells called stem cells. Stem cells are found in both adult tissues and embryonic tissues, and have the ability to change into whatever type of cell is needed and make new generations of those needed cells. Stem cells may soon be a centerpiece in the treatment of degenerative diseases such as Parkinson's or Alzheimers. They may also help treat trauma, blindness, deafness, cardiovascular disease, gastrointestinal disease, diabetes, cancer, arthritis, baldness, and more. Many of the non-hormonal remedies mentioned in this book may also be improved by stem cell treatment. While not yet common practice, I believe that stem cell therapy is the next medical frontier.

ant to insulin, however, blood glucose levels can get too high, which can lead to a number of problems. Insulin resistance is associated with excess weight around the waist, high LDL (bad cholesterol), low HDL (good cholesterol), high levels of triglycerides, and high blood pressure. It can result in heart attacks, strokes, obesity, and diabetes—the top four health problems in the United States today—as well as numerous other health conditions.

To keep insulin resistance from leading to serious health issues, you must focus on exercise and diet. By building more muscle cells and shrinking fat cells through exercise, you can increase insulin sensitivity. (See "Non-Hormonal Ways to Boost Your Metabolism" on page 148.) Moreover, by following a diet that pairs protein with complex carbohydrates like whole grains and vegetables, includes smaller and lighter meals, and excludes refined sugars (such as those found in cake, cookies, and soda), you can maintain a proper level of blood glucose and avoid insulin resistance altogether.

Unfortunately, another type of hormonal resistance seems to go hand in hand with insulin resistance, making it even harder to change your diet. It is called leptin resistance.

Leptin Resistance

Fat is smarter than we think. It has been shown that fat cells actually secrete hormones, one of which is leptin. Leptin is responsible for telling your brain to stop eating because you are full and have enough fat stored already. If you ignore these signals and overeat, fat begins to accumulate in your body. In addition, leptin keeps trying to tell you to stop consuming food, thus increasing its levels. If leptin levels remain high for a long period of time, your brain no longer listens to leptin's message. Consequently, the hypothalamus does not receive signals from leptin and thinks that the body is starving. The hypothalamus then does all it can to hold on to every pound of fat and even encourages you to eat by making you feel hungry. This scenario is called leptin resistance, and studies have shown that most overweight and obese people deal with this problem. And unfortunately, chronically high leptin levels discourage growth hormone production, making it more difficult to stay fit. Leptin resistance could be one of the main reasons why those who are overweight still cannot lose an ounce of fat despite their best efforts.

So what should you do if you think you have leptin resistance? Well, the worst thing you could do is starve yourself. Starvation or low-calorie dieting decreases your metabolic rate significantly and gives only minimal weight-loss results. When you return to eating a normal diet, even if it is healthy, your metabolic rate will be lower than when you started and may not return to its prior level, making it possible to gain back even more weight!

Once you have had a blood test to determine whether or not you are actually leptin resistant, your clinician can devise a treatment plan. Most likely your blood test will reveal that you have insulin resistance along with leptin resistance, so you will need to adopt the appropriate lifestyle changes to manage these conditions. Dietary adjustments play a major role in the treatment of both issues.

Change Your Diet

Preventing insulin and leptin resistance requires a diet that promotes health, longevity, and weight loss. Learning how many calories you require each day is important, but a good diet is not just about counting calories. A good diet also takes into account the types and amounts of food consumed. The following suggestions are the dietary prescription for hormonal balance. They are contrary to Western diet and lifestyle, which promote insulin resistance, cardiovascular problems, and stress at every age. While there are various diets I support for other conditions, the principles discussed here will aid in hormonal balance. But don't think of these tips as just a diet, for the word diet implies a temporary change. Consider them a dietary lifestyle that will stay with you over the long run, keeping you healthy and feeling good.

Avoid Chemicals and High-Fructose Corn Syrup

World War II brought packaged foods and preservatives to the United States. Such foods were well regarded because they allowed for quick stocking of supermarkets across the country and could last a long time in case of famine or emergency. Sixty years later, food companies are still packaging everything under the sun. The problem is that most packaged foods are highly processed and contain refined sugars and chemicals. They have chemical preservatives to maintain freshness as well as manufactured ingredients such as high-fructose corn syrup (HFCS) to make food taste better.

HFCS was created in the 1970s by pressing and genetically altering modified cornstarch into a mixture that contains 55 percent fructose. It tastes sweeter and is cheaper than natural sugar and is found in baked goods, sodas, sauces, and lots of other packaged foods. HFCS can raise triglycerides, raising the risk of heart problems and diabetes. According to the US Department of Agriculture, consumption of HFCS increased by more than 1000 percent between 1970 and 1990. During this time, there was an alarming increase in obesity. Studies suggest that since fructose does not stimulate insulin secretion, the body does not know when it has exceeded its proper sugar intake limit and therefore wants to eat more calories. Additionally, fructose metabolism may favor the synthesis of fat, further adding to the problem.

In addition to the problem of HFCS, the chemicals and pesticides found in food can mimic certain estrogenic processes, which can lead to a variety of serious health issues. But how do you avoid HFCS, chemical, and pesticides when almost every food contains one or more of these substances? First of all, buy organic whole foods that are single ingredients—an apple, rather than an apple-flavored snack bar. Since HFCS and pesticides are not found in nature, a food that claims to be organic cannot contain these chemicals. If you do not have access to organic fruits and vegetables, buy natural cleansing agents that remove pesticides. When it comes to meat, look for free-range, grass-fed, and organic options.

Shop the perimeter of a supermarket—the produce and meat sections—and avoid the middle part of the store, where the frozen foods, packaged chips, and cookies are found. The dairy and bakery sections should be visited with caution. Many baked goods contain HFCS and most dairy products come from cows that have been given antibiotics and fed rBGH, an artificial bovine growth hormone that increases milk output.

Choose the Right Fats

Fat is an essential part of a diet because every cell is coated with it. Your body can't make essential fatty acids omega-3 and omega-6, so they must be consumed. Omega-3 fatty acids are found in cold-water fish (salmon, sardines, mackerel, black cod, herring, and bluefish), walnuts, and flaxseeds. The body uses omega-3 fatty acids to help build hormones, minimize inflammation, and balance blood clotting and cell growth. They have also been shown to prevent coronary heart disease and strengthen the immune system. Omega-6 fatty acids, which are found in most nuts, seeds, and refined oils (the main oil in packaged snack and fast foods), promote inflammation when eaten in excess. Years ago, both types of fatty acids were typically consumed in proper proportions. Modern Western culture, however, now ingests much more of the omega-6 fatty acids relative to omega-3s, as most foods in the Western diet are abundant in omega-6s but lack omega-3s. The ratio of omega-6 to omega-3 in the common modern diet is 15 to 1. This skewed ratio may contribute to obesity, depression, dyslexia, hyperactivity, cancer, and even a tendency toward violence.

While saturated fat has been regarded as bad for some time now, in recent years, trans fats have proven to be even worse. Trans fats are the result of commercial hydrogenation of vegetable oils. These fats permanently attach to heart muscle. Eating 5 g of trans fat per day increases heart disease risk by 25 percent. In addition to posing cardiovascular problems, excess trans fats are carcinogenic.

About 30 percent of your total daily calories can come from fat, but most of the fat you consume should be monounsaturated and polyunsaturated. To promote longevity, the ratio of omega-6 to omega-3 fatty acids in the diet should be about 2 to 1. Limit saturated fats to less than 7 percent, and avoid trans fats completely. You can find monounsaturated fats in avocados and nuts—especially walnuts, cashews, almonds, and nut butters made from these nuts. Wild salmon, sardines, black cod, omega-3 fortified eggs, flaxseed, and fish-oil supplements are excellent sources of omega-3 fatty acids. Saturated fat intake may be reduced by eating less butter, cheese, cream, full-fat dairy products, skins of chicken and turkey, and fatty red meats like lamb and beef.

Stay away from genetically modified (GMO) safflower and sunflower oils, corn oil, cottonseed oil, and mixed vegetable oils. Strictly exclude all products made with partially hydrogenated oils (trans fats) of any kind, including margarine and vegetable shortening. Instead, cook with extra-virgin olive oil, organic canola oil, or coconut oil. Coconut oil, while high in saturated fat, contains medium-chain triglycerides that the body uses efficiently for fuel. Numerous studies suggest that the non-hydrogenated version of this oil may help promote a feeling of fullness and weight loss.

Eat Smaller Amounts More Frequently

When you eat certain foods or when you eat excessive amounts, glucose and insulin levels spike rapidly, contributing over time to obesity and diabetes. Therefore, it is best to eat the kinds and portions of foods that do not spike your blood sugar and subsequently your insulin. Also remember that extreme highs and lows put stress on the body, which spikes your cortisol level, promoting belly fat in the process.

A portion usually contains 200 to 300 calories. You may wonder how you can get through the day! But the body runs best when you constantly feed it small amounts. You may have heard the advice to eat five small meals a day instead of three big ones. This is so sugar and insulin levels do not rise and then plummet, but instead stay fairly stable. Your metabolism stays revved up throughout the day, and your chance of developing insulin resistance decreases.

Always Pair Protein with Carbohydrates

As the Zone Diet advocates, it is important to pair protein with carbohydrates in a particular ratio at each main meal. (And when you choose carbohydrates, opt for complex carbs, such as whole grains and legumes, instead of simple carbs, like candy and soda, which spike blood sugar levels much more dramatically.) Essentially, for every 2 g of carbohydrate, you need 1 g of protein. (Amounts of fiber and sugar alcohols should be subtracted from the total grams of carbohydrates.) So, for example, let's say your meal contains 22 g of carbohydrates, 7 g of fiber, and 2 g of sugar alcohols. The net carb balance is 22 g minus 9 g, or 11 g. Therefore, you need 5.5 g of protein (half the amount of carbs) to balance the sugar load. Vegetables (except for corn and potatoes) in any portion may be added.

Some carbohydrate-protein pairings are obvious, others not so much. There will be some foods you won't want to give up, and you probably won't have to. There are many delicious ways to meet your meal requirements. For example, you may enjoy steel-cut oats made with unsweetened soy milk in the morning. If you are allergic to both soy and dairy milks, try almond milk instead. Since it has much less protein in it, you can stir in vanilla-flavored protein powder to the milk before heating the oats (avoid heating the oats in the microwave; use the stove top instead) to keep your ratio in balance. You can even add a dash of cinnamon for flavor and a few walnuts to add more calories and omega-3 fats to the meal.

For lunch, try an open-faced tuna melt. Use one whole-grain bread slice, and pile on tuna salad—a mixture of tuna, celery, onion, capers, seasonings, white pepper, a dash of Himalayan sea salt, fresh lemon juice, and olive oil. Consider topping it with grilled bell peppers or tomatoes. You can even sprinkle it with a bit of low-fat or vegan cheddar cheese. Heat the tuna melt under the broiler for a few minutes. The sandwich will contain about 20 g of carbs and 18 g of protein, with about 200 calories. Add a small bunch of grapes for dessert (about 14 g of carbs and 50 calories) to make a perfectly balanced and satisfying meal!

Snack

Most people think of snacks as bad, but the right snacks can actually be good for you! Snacks help maintain correct levels of serotonin—the neurotransmitter in the brain that calms mood, makes you feel happy, promotes satiety, helps manage junk food cravings, and aids in melatonin and estrogen production. Levels of serotonin in the brain can dip with age, stress, and during menopause. Winter can lower them even further. Unfortunately, a low-carbohydrate or low-calorie diet also depletes serotonin and depresses thyroid function. This is why the Atkins Diet and other high-protein and low-carbohydrate diets are not a lifestyle but only short-lived fads. The trick to snacking on carbs is to choose ones that don't spike insulin and don't require protein pairing, which include fruits such as apples, apricots, cherries, grapefruit, nectarines, peaches, pears, and plums.

Eat Vegetables and Fruit

Vegetables are complex carbohydrates and most do not spike blood glucose. They may be eaten in unlimited quantities, regardless of protein eaten. Eating at least eight portions of vegetables each day will provide your body with vital nutrients and fiber. Starchy vegetables, however, such as corn or potatoes, are carbohydrates that must be paired with protein to prevent sugar spikes in the blood.

In addition to vegetables, eat three servings of fresh fruit every day, but be sure to opt for fruits that don't spike insulin levels. A single apple, four apricots, fourteen cherries, half of a grapefruit, a lemon, a lime, a nectarine, a peach, a pear, or two plums are all appropriate choices and serving sizes. The fiber content in these fruits delays the sugar absorption into the blood. To get the fiber, though, be sure to eat the skins (not the rinds). These fruits should be your mid-morning and mid-afternoon snack to encourage serotonin production without spiking insulin. All other fruits produce insulin spikes and should be paired with protein.

Go Vegetarian

A vegetarian or vegan diet is an excellent lifestyle to maintain wellness and health (and hormonal balance), but for many westerners, it is too radical or unappealing. Additionally, if you are a vegetarian or vegan, it may be too difficult to follow the diet prescription previously outlined. Nuts, seeds, and legumes are good sources of protein, but often cannot stand up to the high-carbohydrate loads of a vegetarian or vegan diet. If you avoid animal products but would like to incorporate more protein into your diet, seek out a veggie protein powder supplement. There are veggie protein products that contain a blend of pea, hemp, and organic rice proteins. This combination provides all the essential amino acids needed to build muscle.

Drink Water

Drink water to stay hydrated. A glass of water has a way of making us feel full. Water is calorie-free, helps the kidneys clean the blood, and hydrates cells. Try to drink from distilled and filtered sources, because tap water can contain unhealthy chemicals and minerals like lead, radon, and nitrates. How much you need to drink depends on your activity level, diet, and environment. To stay hydrated, it is best to drink small amounts throughout the day, rather than large jugs of water only a few times a day. The body cannot absorb large quantities of liquid at one time, so you will find yourself repeatedly going to the bathroom.

To reduce the risk of osteoporosis, stay away from soda and other acidic carbonated beverages containing phosphorous. Acidity and excess phosphorous will prevent calcium absorption and leech manganese and calcium from bone. Obviously, soda should also be avoided because of its HFCS content and calorie count. Regarding diet soda, studies are progressively showing that they too should be reduced or eliminated. Diet soda can promote hunger, which might result in weight gain. Moreover, the chemicals in diet soda have been linked to an increased risk of stroke. Try to limit your intake to less than one diet drink a day or preferably none at all.

Interestingly, oolong and green teas have been shown to increase metabolism and curb hunger. Actually, any warm liquid consumed before a meal will usually curb your appetite. The warm liquid stretches the muscles of the stomach, which signals the brain that there is something in the stomach already, lowering the need for a large amount of food.

Stay Alkaline

The American diet, consisting mainly of processed carbohydrates and fats, promotes an acidic pH in the body. Numerous enzymes and certain hormones such as insulin cannot work efficiently in an acidic environment. In addition, yeast tends to grow in the body when it is too acidic, leading to more yeast infections and intestinal problems. Other issues, including osteoporosis and gingivitis, also thrive in acidic environments.

To promote a more alkaline (basic) pH, consume more fruit and vegetables, limit consumption of processed products, reduce intake of animal fats, and consume lemon juice or organic apple cider vinegar thirty minutes before meals (or use it as a salad dressing). There are some expensive dietary supplements to promote an alkaline pH, but I prefer to promote pH balance through whole foods—save your money for something else. As an added bonus, apple cider vinegar has been shown to promote insulin sensitivity.

Investigate Food Intolerances

Just about everyone has trouble tolerating some foods. You don't have to be clinically allergic to a food to be intolerant of it. Intolerance may develop over years of consuming a particular food in excess or if you have any type of digestive imbalance. Typically, we are intolerant to the foods we love most. This may be because food sensitivities create inflammation, and inflammation leads to a surge of endorphins in the body, which produce soothing effect. You feel good, so you reach for those foods more often. When the body is sensitive to a certain food, it also limits the digestion of nutrients and causes increased fat storage. Food sensitivities can cause weight gain, abdominal bloating, and swelling of the hands, feet, ankles, chin, and eye area. Other possible symptoms include headache, depression, canker sores, chronic sinus congestion or bronchitis, indigestion or heartburn, fatigue, joint pain or arthritis, and diarrhea or constipation.

An elimination diet is the best way to identify which food is causing the problem. The most common dietary intolerances are dairy, gluten, eggs, and nuts. Soy and corn are high on the list, too.

Try Supplements

Thankfully, there are a number of supplements that may help you decrease insulin resistance and avoid even more serious health issues down the road. If you are insulin resistant or predisposed to this health problem, the following substances can be added to your daily routine in the specified dosages:

- **Alpha Lipoic Acid (ALA).** The main function of ALA is to burn glucose, but it also maintains collagen in the skin, is a powerful antioxidant, increases your levels of vitamins C and E, raises your coenzyme Q_{10} and glutathione levels, stops the inflammatory and immunologic response to cardiovascular artery disease, prevents cataracts, and has many more functions. While found in spinach, meat, and potatoes, it is impossible to obtain ALA in sufficient quantities from the diet, so it should be supplemented. Take 200 to 300 mg a day. (Be aware that 600 mg a day may decrease the active thyroid hormone available in the body, resulting in hypothyroidism.)

- **Biotin.** Biotin is needed by the body to metabolize carbohydrates and control blood sugar levels. Take 4 to 8 mg a day.

- **Chromium Picolinate.** Among other benefits, this substance minimizes cravings, makes insulin more effective at lowering blood sugar, and helps with fat loss by burning calories and increasing endurance. It is naturally abundant in broccoli. A high-carbohydrate diet, vitamin C, injury, and routine exercise will deplete chromium in the body. Take 400 to 600 mcg a day to treat insulin resistance, or 200 to 300 mcg a day to fight sugar cravings.

- **Coenzyme Q_{10}.** This supplement helps prevent insulin levels from elevating in the blood. Take 50 to 300 mg a day. Formulations of coenzyme Q_{10} are more effective if suspended in oil.

- **Conjugated Linoleic Acid (CLA).** CLA is a fatty acid with powerful metabolic effects. It promotes weight loss and helps with insulin sensitivity. Take 100 to 500 mg to prevent insulin resistance or 2,000 mg to treat it. You can also take 3,000 to 4,000 mg a day to promote weight loss.

- **Fiber.** Fiber helps slow digestion and prevents blood sugar from spiking shortly after a meal. Soluble fiber is particularly important to people with insulin resistance, as it helps slow insulin's response to a rise in blood sugar and helps them lose weight because it makes them feel fuller. Make an effort to get 30 to 50 g of fiber every day.

- **Magnesium.** Magnesium plays many roles in the body, one of which is to increase insulin sensitivity. High stress, certain prescription drugs, diarrhea, injury, and excessive intake of sugar, caffeine, alcohol, soda, trans fats, or fiber are just some of the reasons behind a depletion of magnesium. Dietary sources include nuts, seeds, grains, soy, leafy greens, grains, avocados, and dried fruit. If your diet is lacking in these foods, supplement with 600 to 800 mg a day.

- **Manganese.** Abnormal metabolism of glucose has been correlated to a lack of manganese. Dietary sources include whole grains, avocados, and seaweed. Daily manganese supplements of 5 to 10 mg may be taken.

- **Omega-3 Fatty Acids.** In addition to slowing the absorption of carbs in the blood, it also prevents and relieves inflammatory conditions (like arthritis); lowers triglycerides, total cholesterol, LDL, and blood pressure; breaks up blood clots; improves memory and focus; alleviates depression and psychosis; and reduces the risk of certain cancers. Take 1 to 6 g a day, and choose fish oil supplements that contain both EPA and DHA.

- **Taurine.** If possible, take a serum amino acid test to see if you need taurine supplementation. Taurine is an amino acid that requires zinc for activity and can be depleted by chronic stress. It promotes glucose metabolism and improves sensitivity to insulin. If needed, take 1,000 to 3,000 mg a day.

- **Vanadium.** This mineral helps improve insulin sensitivity, may prevent insulin resistance, and reduces the risk of developing diabetes. Take 25 to 50 mg a day.

- **Vitamin B Complex.** Refined and simple sugar consumption causes the overproduction of insulin. When there is a lack of B vitamins, the body is unable to harness the enzyme needed to metabolize sugar into energy. Supplement with 50 to 100 mg a day.

- **Vitamin C.** This vitamin helps improve insulin sensitivity and can also restore the function of cells that line the arteries in those with cardiovascular problems. Take 1,000 to 3,000 mg a day.

- **Vitamin E.** Among other benefits, high doses of vitamin E help improve insulin sensitivity in overweight people. Supplement with 600 to 1,200 IU a day.

- **Zinc.** In vitro studies show that insulin interacts with zinc, increasing the binding ability of insulin to its receptor. As such, insulin sensitivity can improve after supplementation with zinc. Take 25 to 50 mg a day.

Always be sure to buy pharmaceutical-grade products by trusted manufacturers when choosing supplements. And always tell your physician which supplements you wish to try (and at which dosages), as new information regarding the benefits and side effects of these substances is released frequently and you should remain informed.

How to Maintain Your New Dietary Lifestyle

You cannot change the way you eat overnight and expect to remain faithful to such a drastic lifestyle overhaul. The transition to a new dietary plan should be undertaken over the course of a few weeks instead. Along the way, there are many ways to make the adjustment easier and more successful.

Get Support

Ask your friends and family for their support. If you can get one of them to make some changes, too, you will be much more successful than if you do it alone. Persuading your family to change might be easier than you think. If you happen to be the one in the house who already cooks dinner for the family, you get to choose what is on the menu anyway.

Meditate

Visualization or meditation can help. To begin, lie on your back in a dark room and close your eyes. Concentrate on your breathing until you are relaxed and then repeat an encouraging phrase such as "I love healthy foods." (Don't pick a negative phrase like "I hate cookies and ice cream.") If you find your mind wandering, focus on your breathing again. You can practice meditation for as little as five minutes a day, if that's all the time you have to spare.

Find Time to Cook

Since most healthful foods aren't found in packages or at restaurants, you will have to start preparing your own meals. This means you will need to make a balanced breakfast, take a lunch and healthy snacks to work, and have a good home-cooked dinner most days of the week. Therefore, you must find time to go grocery shopping fairly often and prepare these daily meals.

Discover Healthy Recipes

Search for recipes that you find tasty as well as healthy. If you have a culinary flair, try to come up with your own recipes. Modify an unhealthy meal into a healthy one. For example, a cheeseburger with French fries can become an organic ground turkey breast (hold the bun) with avocado and a garden salad with apples and walnuts. Try not to splurge, but don't obsess over it if you do. A few hundred calories are not going to make you fat, but chronic overeating will.

Once you've found some delicious recipes, take the time to enjoy them. Sit down at the table and spend a good thirty minutes eating your meal. Do not rush. Savor the flavors!

Keep a Food Diary

It is easy to tell yourself that you eat healthfully. But do you really? Did you forget about that fun-size Snickers bar you sneaked in? How about that latte? The only way you can be straight about what you put in your body is to log your food intake. This practice is especially important during the transition into a new dietary lifestyle. You may be surprised by all the calories that can make their way into your body throughout the day.

Two weeks before committing to your new lifestyle, write down all foods and drinks you consume, as well as how you felt physically, emotionally, and mentally before and after you consumed them. This might pinpoint the times of day that you are vulnerable to certain cravings. When you start your new lifestyle, maintain your food diary and mark how you feel after making healthier choices. After a couple of weeks into the new lifestyle, you will be getting used to eating healthfully. When you look back through the log, you will notice how much better you feel physically and emotionally.

NON-HORMONAL WAYS TO BOOST YOUR METABOLISM

If you're over forty years of age, you know how difficult it can be to maintain your body. Parts of it start drooping or expanding even when you eat sensibly. The best way to defy gravity and battle the bulge is to increase your metabolism by building up and working out your muscles, which are the secret to boosting your metabolism and fat-burning potential. Muscle cells use more energy than any other type of cell, so the more muscle you have, the higher your metabolism. The higher your metabolism, the more energy you require from foods to maintain your weight.

Lose Fat, Not Muscle

When you lose a pound, you don't lose just fat, but also some muscle because the body doesn't have to work as hard to carry that extra pound of weight around. As a rule of thumb, if you were to lose ten pounds of body weight, one of those pounds would be muscle. In other words, if you lose weight, your muscle mass will decrease as well, lowering your metabolism. Your ultimate goal should include both fat loss and an increase in muscle mass if you want to keep your metabolism high.

Building muscle requires weight-bearing exercise, like lifting free weights. Burning fat requires low-intensity exercise, like going for a brisk walk. Fat-burning exercise should not be confused with cardiovascular exercise, which requires high energy expenditure (running, swimming, or biking). While cardio conditions your heart and keeps your arteries clean, it burns sugar and muscle before it burns fat. During high-intensity exercise, the body metabolizes nutrients in a certain order: alcohol, carbohydrates, muscle, and finally fat. When you engage in a high-intensity activity such as running, you burn the sugar stored in your muscles first. When the sugar is burned up, you start burning your own muscle, leading to a lower metabolism. Have you ever noticed that long-distance runners have little muscle on their bodies? This is because they burn their own muscle to go the long distance!

So how do you burn fat first? How do you prevent burning your muscle? Imagine that you want to make a pot roast in a crock-pot. Before you head to work, you put the roast in the pot, add a few spices and veggies, add broth, turn on the crock-pot, and head out. When you return eight or nine hours later, the roast is not burned; rather, it is tender, lean, and perfectly cooked. This is because cooking meat at a low heat for an extended period of time will melt the fat off. The slow-cooking method prevents the meat (muscle) from burning. You exercise smarter when you are like the crock-pot, not the high-heat barbeque. If you can keep your fire on low (not off and not too high), you can burn fat all day long!

Know Your Fat-Burning Range

Because each person's metabolism and chemistry are different, each person has a specific fat-burning heart-rate range. In order to burn fat, you must stay within your particular fat-burning range during exercise. While you may learn your fat-burning heart rate with the help of your physician, you may also estimate it on your own by following a few simple calculations. Calculate your maximum heart rate, which equals 220 minus your age. The lower limit of your fat-burning heart rate is your maximum heart rate times 0.55, while the upper limit of your fat-burning heart rate is your maximum heart rate times 0.65. Monitoring your heart rate is essential to staying within the desired zone throughout the day. A digital heart monitor can let you know when you've reached your fat-burning zone.

A comprehensive fitness plan includes living in your fat-burning zone, doing interval training, and engaging in weight-bearing exercise. To achieve and maintain weight loss, the goal is to work out for one hour every day five or six times a week. (When starting this new lifestyle, of course, you must work up to this level of intensity and frequency.)

Live in Your Fat-Burning Zone

If you could keep your heart consistently beating within the fat-burning rate range, you would (with persistence) widen that range so that eventually you would burn fat by engaging in very light activities. You can do any type of movement you like (walking all day long, lifting your legs repeatedly under your desk at work, or going up the stairs every couple of minutes) as long as it gets your heart rate within your unique fat-burning zone.

Trying to stay in your fat-burning zone should be a goal, but it is not the end-all solution to weight loss. You should also supplement with other exercises, because the fat-burning zone does not burn very many total calories unless you are within your range for many hours at a time. Let's say you burn 5 calories per minute while in your fat-burning zone, 3 of which are fat calories. If you are able to do this for about two hours a day, you will burn 360 fat calories that day. Since a reduction of 3,500 calories is required to lose a pound of body weight, it would take about ten days to lose a pound of body fat, which may sound discouraging to you. Meanwhile, you will inevitably lose some muscle as well, decreasing your metabolism. This explains why living in your fat-burning zone is not enough on its own. You also need to weight train, be mindful of calories, and engage in a few vigorous physical activities.

Add High-Intensity Interval Training

Some studies have shown that metabolism is increased by doing ten repetitions of a high-intensity activity followed by a short recovery period. For example, a person could sprint for sixty seconds, walk for one minute, and repeat this cycle ten times. In twenty minutes or less, interval training can jump start resting metabolism for the next twenty-four hours. Unlike a steady workout such as distance running, during which your body begins conserving energy, the ever-changing pace tricks the body, making it unable to identify a stable pattern. So, even though endurance cardio burns more calories than a shorter session of interval training, the interval training will produce more fat loss over the following hours.

What's the best way to figure out your heart range for the intense part of the interval? Typically you take 220 minus your age, and then take 80 percent of that value as the heart rate you should maintain during high-intensity exercise. High-intensity workouts, however, should be done with caution. If you have a heart condition or are in poor general health, you need permission from your doctor to train in this manner. If you are not in shape, you should take the time to build up to this level of exercise, and you should talk to your health care provider before beginning. At first, you may get through only three or four cycles. Keep it up, and the number of cycles you can do will increase by the week.

Don't engage in interval-training two days in a row. Give your muscles a chance to recover. You should have a light carbohydrate snack (a piece of fruit, for example) before each session. Eat protein (or have a protein shake) within thirty minutes after each session. The carbohydrate will provide your muscles with energy (glucose), while the protein will allow your body to repair and build your muscles.

Pump Iron

As previously mentioned, the main way to increase metabolism is to build more muscle. Since muscle uses far more energy than any other cell in the body, the more muscle you have, the higher your metabolism. To build muscle, you need weight-lifting exercises. As a bonus, such exercises also slow osteoporosis progression.

The first step in weight training is to find a gym with weight-lifting machines and free weights. Learn how to use the gym equipment and how to hold and lift free weights without hurting yourself. Once you know proper form, you can plan a routine. This is best done by working with a personal trainer. Next, weight train for thirty minutes to an hour, at least three days a week You must think of these sessions as important appointments that you cannot miss (like your job). Do not weight train on the days that you do interval work. This ensures that your muscles recover from the intervals, which are very taxing. If you must weight lift on the same day as the intervals, you should give yourself at least an eight-hour break between these two exercises.

When choosing the amount of weight for an exercise, the rule of thumb is to be able to do about twelve to fifteen repetitions before your muscles are exhausted and need a break. If you are worried about getting too bulky, use lighter weights and do more repetitions.

It is hard to stay motivated when working out alone. Taking a "body pump" or circuit-training class at your local gym will provide you with a comprehensive muscle workout. These types of classes guide you through various weight-bearing or resistance exercises for thirty to sixty minutes without much recovery time between sets. This allows you to work most of your body's muscle groups. Often these classes also provide an aerobic workout, depending on the pace and intensity.

Bulk Up Before You Slim Down

Some people find that their bodies get bigger when they incorporate weight training into an exercise regimen, so they quit the weight training and focus on cardio exercise instead. Cardio, while heart healthy, promotes the burning of muscle and sugar rather than fat, which can lower your metabolism and prevent further fat loss. Some of the most heart-healthy people are chubby and have low metabolisms because they are busy doing too much cardio and neglecting their muscles.

When you do muscle-building exercise, you actually cause tiny tears in your muscle fibers which make room for more muscle fibers to appear. This is essentially how the body builds more muscle on top of existing muscle. But, as you may well know, the day after you work those muscles with weights, you feel sore. This is due in part to the tearing of your muscles and the build-up of lactic acid and other metabolites during your workout. Tearing causes inflammation and swelling, so it is necessary to stay hydrated before, during, and well after your weight training to help flush out these inflammatory factors. It is also a good idea to incorporate antioxidants such as vitamin C, E, and A, glutathione, coenzyme Q_{10}, selenium, lycopene, flavonoids, and lignans, or natural anti-inflammatory agents such as turmeric, curcumin, ginger, shitake or maitake mushrooms, green tea, and broccoli, into your post-workout meal. Talk to your doctor about using pharmaceutical anti-inflammatory drugs such as ibuprofen or other agents like it, especially if you take blood thinners. It is also not a good idea to self-treat chronic inflammation with ibuprofen without talking to your physician.

Women tend to gain muscle more quickly than they lose fat. This is worth remembering if you are a woman who is starting weight training. While you might have been told that muscle is denser and more compact than fat tissue, you will inevitably notice an increase in body mass if you pack on muscle without losing fat or if you are swollen. If you keep up your weight training, however, your muscle mass will soon cause your fat to melt away, revealing a svelte figure.

Stretch and Work Your Core

Ballet dancers have long, lean figures. The combination of extensive stretching, posture training, cardio, and light weight training yields a dancer's body. Of course, a professional dancer works very hard and dances most days of the week for hours at a time, but you can still gain valuable tips from such training.

First, it is important to stretch your muscles before and after you work them out. Stretching at least five to ten minutes both before and after a workout can prevent injury. It also creates a leaner and longer figure. If you find your muscles still appear bulky or bunched, try massaging the muscle group on a regular basis.

Working on your posture can also promote a long and lean look. Certain yoga and Pilates classes focus on strengthening core muscles (those that hold up the torso and body). Maintaining a strong core is a great step toward having correct posture. Some personal trainers recommend working on your core heavily in the beginning stages of building your new body. The thought behind this is that the core is the body's foundation, similar to a foundation of a house. Without a solid foundation, the house is not sturdy and will fall. Similarly, without a strong core, you may injure yourself more often. Taking a Pilates class will help strengthen your core muscles.

Do Some Cardio

If you had to run for your life, could you? Actually, running and other exercises that increase your heart rate *can* save your life. They're the best way to maintain your cardiovascular system and prevent coronary heart disease, congestive heart failure, and other heart diseases. In addition to burning a lot of calories, working out your heart on a regular basis will also increase the rate of your metabolism over time.

You've learned that constant high-intensity training like cardio burns sugar calories first, and then muscle, all before fat. While not ideal for weight loss, cardio is important for your overall health. Cardio does burn up a lot of calories, including some fat calories.

Therefore, cardio should be done at least three days a week for thirty minutes at a time. Doing cardio properly is all about staying within the cardio target heart-rate zone. Calculate your cardio heart-rate zone by subtracting your age from 220 and then multiplying that number by 60 to 80 percent. For example, if you were a fifty-five-year-old woman, the low end of your cardio target heart rate would be 99 beats per minute. In other words, 220 minus 55 equals 165, and 165 times 0.6 is 99. Your upper limit would be 132, or 165 times 0.8. Staying within this range for cardio workouts would safely work your heart and cardiovascular system.

Cardiovascular training doesn't have to involve running; it can be swimming, biking, jumping rope, dancing, kick boxing, or whatever you like that keeps your heart rate within 60 to 80 percent of its maximum capacity. Never overexert yourself to the point of chest pain, though. Start out with thirty minutes, two to three times a week. You can alternate your interval days with your cardio days to allow for proper muscle regeneration. Combining these two forms of training with weight-bearing exercise will have you looking like your fit self in about twelve weeks.

Follow a Program

A good fitness program includes intervals, cardiovascular training, weight lifting, and fat-burning exercise. In a decent fitness regimen, four hours a week are spent on physical activity. Intervals are done three days a week for twenty minutes each session, and cardio and weight training are done for thirty minutes three times a week. Both cardio and intervals must be done in addition to weight-bearing exercise. During cardio, the heart beat is consistently kept between 60 and 80 percent of maximum. Intervals cause the heart rate to fluctuate, increasing metabolism for the following twenty-four hours. Since intervals are very intense, muscles should be rested for twelve to twenty-four hours before doing any weight training or other vigorous exercise.

The following table lists a weekly exercise plan that can be incorporated into your life with just a little effort. It only takes four hours a week to do, and will provide you with invaluable health benefits.

As you surely noticed, Sunday is a full day off. And, although it is not listed, fat-burning exercise, such as a brisk walk, should

WEEKLY EXERCISE PLAN						
EXERCISE	Monday	Tuesday	Wednesday	Thursday	Friday	Saturday
High-Intensity Interval Training	20 Minutes	Off	20 Minutes	Off	20 Minutes	Off
Cardio	Off	30 Minutes	Off	30 Minutes	Off	30 Minutes
Weights	Off	30 Minutes	Off	30 Minutes	Off	30 Minutes
Total	20 Minutes	1 Hour	20 Minutes	1 Hour	20 Minutes	1 Hour

be performed throughout each day (even Sunday). Fat-burning exercises can drastically add to the total hours of physical activity performed and fat calories burned per week. It may be ideal to do more fat-burning activities on the days you do intervals, since you work your body for only twenty minutes on those days.

Mix It Up

If you are happy to run on a treadmill for your intervals and cardio training, and always perform the same types of weight training, you will see results, but you may also hit a plateau quickly. A plateau is reached when the rate of result does not happen as rapidly as it did before. This happens when you do the same type of exercise regimen without variation. Mixing up your routines every couple of weeks prevents a plateau.

Let's say that it has been twelve weeks since the start of your new active lifestyle and exercise regimen. During this period, you ran for thirty minutes three times a week and performed interval training by sprinting and then walking over the course of twenty minutes three days a week. You also used gym machines to work your muscles three times a week. You experienced a weight loss of five pounds and a 4-percent decline in body fat. While you are happy with the results, you notice that the last couple of weeks have not seemed very rewarding or motivating because you have hit a plateau. So you decide to take a circuit-training class at the gym as your weight training, jump rope as interval training, and take up kick boxing as your cardio workout. If you switch back and forth from your old routine to your new one every couple of weeks, you should continue to see phenomenal results.

Stay Motivated

Similar to the struggle of following a new diet, sticking to a fitness program at the beginning of a new active lifestyle can be difficult. Thankfully, there are ways to keep up your motivation.

Plan Ahead

When you first start out, make a list of times in your schedule when you can exercise, and then schedule at least two days a week of fitness. Gradually add more days a week, but in the beginning, only schedule as much as you feel you can accomplish. Remember, fitness makes you feel and look younger. As motivation, think of these appointments as anti-aging treatments.

Join a Group

Join a gym or visit your local YMCA, college, or community center that has group classes. There are many local fitness studios and gyms that have group classes and circuit training. You can search online to find local locations. Group fitness ensures that you won't be alone. The presence of other people will motivate you. Group classes are also a great way to make new friends that will support your healthy lifestyle.

Measure Yourself

Before you begin your new fitness program, make sure to measure your fitness statistics (height, weight, waistline, etc). Also test your baseline fitness level. You can have this done by a personal trainer at a gym for a fee. It is important that you know your starting point so you can track your progress over time.

Avoid Workouts During the First Week

During the first week of committing to a fitness program, don't work out at all. Instead, go through the motions of getting ready to work out. For example, put on your fitness clothes, heart rate monitor, and shoes and then take them right off. Do this for one full week each day. Remember, even the simple task of getting ready to exercise has prevented people from exercising entirely. If you can't even put on your gear, then how are you going to commit to a healthy and active lifestyle? Take the first week to get in the right mindset.

Don't Weigh Yourself

After your initial weigh-in, hide your weight scale. Since the optimal fitness program involves not only fat burning but also muscle building, your weight might not drop much or may even increase! You have heard that muscle weighs more than fat, but if you are working out hard and haven't lost even one pound, you will feel discouraged and abandon your fitness regimen. It is better to measure your fitness progress by how your clothes fit and how energetic and happy you feel. Change will happen gradually; be patient. Once you have met your fitness goals and final body weight, it will be important to reintroduce the scale to make sure there are few fluctuations.

Enlist Support

Make sure your family is on board with your new lifestyle. Talk to your spouse or partner about your goals and hopes for a healthy life. State that you need support. Your best friends will be your other advocates in promoting your health. Tell them that you can't make it without their encouragement. You might even inspire some of your loved ones to change their own lives. Maybe one of them will become your new workout partner!

Find a Hobby

If you just can't commit yourself to working out in a gym five or six days a week, consider taking up an active hobby. The hobby can be a Latin dance class with your spouse, tennis with your best friend, golf without the golf cart, synchronized swimming, water volleyball, long walks with your dog, or any other activity that gets you moving. The possibilities are endless, so get creative and make it fun.

Be an Activist

If you have interest in a cause, such as fighting breast cancer or curing autism, become an active voice in that group. You can then organize fundraising events like a walk or dance. This will not only lift your emotional spirit, but also get you fit.

Do the Seemingly Impossible

Commit to something seemingly impossible, like running a 5K or even a marathon. If you are a person who strives to be the best or are ambitious, deciding to run a marathon can be very rewarding not only physically but also mentally. Obviously, it will take a lot of work on your part. You will have to work out consistently and with a trainer or local group, but once you achieve your goal you will feel it was worth the effort. Check your community's website to see when a race is scheduled. Allow at least a few months to work up to that fitness level and go for it!

Use Every Piece of the Puzzle

When followed as closely as possible, the exercise regimen described in this chapter should yield some results by week twelve. You will note some slight difference in your physique by week six, and between weeks six and twelve you will notice more. Physical activity, however, accounts for only 30 percent of the healthy-and-beautiful-body equation. Diet and hormonal balance are also parts of it. If you are not seeing the benefits of exercise, you may need to reevaluate your diet or optimize your hormones. Be patient, stay motivated, and shortly you will start to feel and see the benefits of an active lifestyle.

You might stick to a vigorous regimen for a week and then not be able to keep it up despite all your planning and motivation. Do not get discouraged! Drastically changing a behavior takes months or even years. But if you simply choose one change and try your best to maintain it for a month or two, then you can slowly introduce another to your routine. Remember that a long journey begins with a single step. Within a year, you might wake up one morning to see that you have progressed from a sedentary lifestyle to an active, healthier one.

NON-HORMONAL TREATMENTS FOR STRESS

Your body was designed to use the hormone cortisol to cope with acute extreme stress. But when stress occurs day after day, soon the body's cortisol levels are out of control, with serious repercussions that may include insulin resistance, high blood pressure, or depression. If you have already reached this point, you must adopt a balanced lifestyle that fosters health and happiness.

Humans don't handle long periods of stress very well. Under stress, the body needs many more nutrients and builds up a lot of toxins. These increased demands have to be met, or your health will deteriorate. Dr. James Wilson has been a pioneer in treating chronic stress and adrenal fatigue. The following recommendations, endorsed by Dr. Wilson, help the body resist stress and may be employed during all stages of adrenal dysfunction.

Exercise

Exercise is very important element in stress relief. It boosts metabolism and energy, promotes restful sleep, and eliminates excess toxins. The best time to exercise is in the morning, as it can jumpstart your day. To avoid adding to your stress, do not engage in competitive sports or intense exercise. Anything that agitates your body and mind is best avoided for the time being. The best exercises for stressed-out individuals are fun and energizing ones like swimming, hiking, or dancing. If you are extremely fatigued, try walking briskly with a friend.

Change Your Diet

Fluctuating blood sugar levels are a major source of stress. To avoid this problem, eat regular meals: breakfast by 10 AM, lunch or a snack at noon, a snack mid afternoon, dinner by 6 PM, and an optional small snack before bed. Each main meal should focus on vegetables, protein, and good fats, and less on simple carbohydrates. Don't consume junk food, sugar, caffeine, chocolate, trans fats, or alcohol; these substances tend to spike sugar levels and then let you down quickly. If your diet centers on these empty calories, you will find your energy drops rapidly during mid morning and afternoon, causing you to reach for caffeine or something sweet to drive you.

Don't feel guilty if you want to splurge a little; just schedule your comfort foods in between your main protein-packed meals. Remember, stress increases nutritional demands on the body. Make every calorie count. Mealtimes should be serene and not stressful. Never rush, always eat sitting down, eat with friends or loved ones, chew your food completely, and eat slowly.

Try Supplements to Treat the Effects of Stress

The following supplements are particularly suited to the treatment of stress. This list is a recommended regimen, but your doctor may determine dosages specific to your bodily needs. These amounts should be taken once a day unless otherwise noted:

- Chromium: 200–400 mcg

- Copper: 1–2 mg

- DL-Phenylalanine (DLPA): 500 mg twice a day

- Iodine: 225 mcg

- L-Theanine: 100 mg twice a day

- Magnesium: 400–1,200 mg

- Manganese: 5 mg

- Molybdenum: 50 mcg

- Phosphotidyl Serine: 100 mg three times a day

- S-Adenosyl Methionine (SAMe): 200 mg twice a day

- Selenium: 200–400 mcg

- Vitamin A: 5,000–15,000 IU

- Vitamin B_1: 1.2 mg

- Vitamin B_3: 125–150 mg

- Vitamin B_5: 1,200–1,500 mg

- Vitamin B_6: 150 mg

- Vitamin B_9: 400–800 mcg

- Vitamin B_{12}: 1,000 mcg

- Vitamin C: 2,000–4,000 mg

- Vitamin D_3: 5,000 IU

- Vitamin E: 800 IU

- Zinc: 25 mg

In addition to vitamins, minerals, and amino acids, certain herbs help the body resist stress. They are usually well tolerated and without side effects. Each of the following herbal supplements should be taken at the dosage recommended on its label:

- Ashwagandha

- Rhodiola Rosea Root

- Schizandra Berry Extract

- Siberian Ginseng

- Skullcap Root

- Maca, Holy Basil, Noni, or Reishi Mushroom

As mentioned in regard to vitamins, minerals, and amino acids, you should always let your health care provider know about any herbal supplement regimen you may be considering.

Meditate, Laugh, and Sleep

Meditative acts such as deep breathing, stretching, and yoga are excellent ways to release stress. Meditation can be part of your morning exercise routine, or it can be done during your breaks or at night. A simple meditation program might involve concentrating on breathing in and out while making a conscious effort to relax every muscle in your body. Later, when you master this technique, you can add a phrase to repeat that promotes positive thinking or changes your opinion about a particular matter, such as, "I love my job." If a phrase is repeated enough, you will learn to believe it, and you will change your opinion and behavior. In addition, the simple act of smiling can raise a person's mood. Laughter causes the secretion of endorphins, which can elevate mood as well. Those with chronic stress or adrenal fatigue frequently forget to smile or laugh with loved ones. Make a conscious effort to laugh and smile more often.

Finally, sleep is essential for stress relief and healing. Eight to nine hours of restful sleep is required for both adrenal-fatigued and overly stressed individuals.

Reduce Sources of Stress

One of the most important ways to reduce stress is to recognize that which stresses you out. By taking a good look at your life, you will be able to determine the sources of your stress as well as the changes you can make to eliminate these sources.

Plan Ahead

If you barely make it to work or activities on time, you need to start planning properly. What will it take to get there on time? An extra five minutes? Plan accordingly. Set your morning alarm for five minutes earlier. You'll be surprised what those five minutes can do for your cortisol levels. If you tend to keep every appointment in your head but find yourself overwhelmed or sleepless about upcoming events, get a planner, a phone application, or a computer calendar. You'll never be late or double-booked again. Some planners double as a journal. I like this option, since you can write down your thoughts and feelings (another great way to release stress).

Reevaluate Your Life

For some, even the little things can cause stress. But will the world come to an end if you don't get to a party or a department store sale? You need to train yourself to put life into perspective. This change is the hardest to master but perhaps the most important to your health and a successful life. I challenge you to decide what matters most in life and start living accordingly. I bet you'll find that money, beauty, perfection, and professional status are at the bottom and love, friendship, happiness, and health are at the top. That's not to say that you should quit your job or not strive for a promotion—just try to find the right balance to lead a happy life. Reevaluating life will be enlightening, and you'll find that you won't stress about the little things as much.

Reevaluate Your Work

Too many tasks and too little time (or skill) to complete them: This is the perfect recipe for stress at work. If your work is the center of your stress, ask yourself why, and then make a plan to address these issues. If there are too many demands and not enough rewards, ask your manager to clarify what is expected of your position. If the hours are too long, ask to change your schedule or take more time off. If you feel stress because you lack a skill, get trained.

Your health is more important than a job. If you spend most of your waking hours at work, you'd better like what you do and with whom you do it. No, I'm not advising you to quit your job today; I'm challenging you to rethink what you want out of life.

Reevaluate Your Money

Debt can be caused by a lack of priorities, not just lack of money. Set your financial and life priorities and create a plan to pay down debts and live within your means. You may choose to have a less fancy car or to rent instead of own. If you are behind in payments, talk to your creditors and negotiate the amount owed.

Reevaluate the People in Your Life

Who are the people who drain the energy from your life? Rank them from least to most severe and brainstorm how you can limit your exposure to them or resolve the conflicts with them. Set a comfortable time limit to confront each issue. Start with the least severe example. Afterward, make a note of the outcome or resolution attained.

On the other hand, spend more time with people who boost your mood and energy. Make a plan and stick to it. Rekindle fading friendships and maintain contact with your circle of loved ones. Make time to pick up the phone and call. Plan a visit. Also remember to express thanks to those you love and those who have helped you.

Heal Adrenal Fatigue

If you already have adrenal fatigue, in addition to the stress-support measures recently outlined, you will need to make some other changes to your daily life in order to regain proper adrenal function.

Sleep Until 9 AM

As you know, sleep is essential to the process of healing and repairing the body. A good night's sleep of at least eight hours can promote a sense of well-being and decrease stress. Those with adrenal fatigue will find that the most restful period of sleep is between 8 and 9 AM. This is why, if you must wake at 7 AM for work, you find yourself hitting the snooze button in the morning. Therefore, you must sleep until 9 AM. If you think you will lose your job by asking to start your work day a little later than usual, get a doctor's note for your employer. Once you have your adrenals working again, you won't need these hours to feel rested.

Get Up on the Right Side of the Bed

Once you are ready to wake, do not leave your bed until you have thought about something positive. Often those with adrenal fatigue suffer from depression and can't find a reason to get out of bed. You must stop this self-destructive thinking and contemplate the happy things in life: your family and friends, an upcoming vacation, fond memories, the smell of a forest, or whatever puts a good feeling in your heart.

Avoid Potassium-Rich Foods in the Morning

People with adrenal fatigue often have an electrolyte imbalance: too much potassium, not enough sodium. Certain diuretics, potassium chloride, and other cardiovascular medications (ACE inhibitors) may also cause this imbalance. Eating fruits that are rich in potassium further increases this imbalance, so avoid bananas, dates, raisins, and figs. In fact, if you crave something salty, don't be afraid to spike your water with a pinch of Himalayan sea salt in the morning or when you are feeling exhausted. You may not realize it, but you probably require salt, so give the body what it wants. But remember to talk to a doctor first if you have a heart condition that restricts you from getting too much salt in your diet.

Rest

You should take two breaks during the day. They should be about fifteen minutes long, and you should spend them lying down (not sitting). Your cortisol dips even lower around 10 AM and 3 PM.

You should take breaks at these times and avoid reaching for processed sugar or caffeine. If you must, lie down in your office or car. Make sure to turn your cell phone off, maybe play soft music, have some tea, or just relax. A doctor's note might make these necessities easier to explain to your manager.

Supplement with Licorice

Licorice root keeps cortisol from being inactivated in the body and also keeps adrenal receptors sensitive to cortisol. It is typically used in the resistant and exhaustion stages of adrenal dysfunction to help increase or maintain proper cortisol levels. Over-the-counter licorice root extract (with a 12-percent glycyrrhizin concentration) may be supplemented at a dosage of 75 to 450 mg a day until adrenal fatigue is remedied. Those with high blood pressure should use it with caution, as licorice root extract will further raise blood pressure over time.

CONCLUSION

If you are not a candidate for systemic hormone therapy, you still have many options in the treatment of symptoms and conditions often associated with menopause and aging. Keep in mind, however, that pharmaceuticals typically do not address the root of these problems; rather, they only mask some of their symptoms. A healthy lifestyle is the foundation of health and wellness. Moreover, natural supplements can help reverse or alleviate many of the symptoms that may be affecting you right now.

Conclusion

While you may understand the importance of keeping fit as you age, I guarantee that you will not run even one mile or lift one weight if your reproductive glands have stopped functioning properly, your adrenals have quit on you, or your pancreas and thyroid aren't working optimally. You may recognize the role of a healthy diet in your life, but I also bet that there is no way you are going to maintain healthy eating habits if your hormone levels aren't right. You'll reach for cookies, lattes, or chocolate to comfort your feeling of depleted energy and depressed mood, which, ironically, only worsen these symptoms. The fact is that getting healthy and feeling good starts with balancing your hormones—all of them. This entails having your hormones tested and supplementing individual hormones when warranted.

I believe that life often gets better after fifty. You know who you are and you're not afraid to be yourself. But if you are feeling unwell due to hormonal imbalance, this problem could be holding you back from a good life. For this reason, it is vital that you know about bioidentical hormone replacement therapy. By now, you understand the many ways in which your hormone levels affect your health, energy, and stress levels. Working toward optimal levels and restoring balance to your hormones will help you lose weight, have more energy, feel better, and enjoy life. And bioidentical hormone replacement therapy can help you achieve these goals safely.

You have the power to change your body and transform your life. With the guidance and encouragement of a health professional who is knowledgeable in bioidentical hormone replacement therapy, the principles you have learned from this book, a strong sense of dedication to your plan, a positive attitude, and the support of your loved ones, you will feel whole again.

About the Author

Amy Lee Hawkins, Pharm.D, is the CEO of Pharm-D Partners, Inc. and founder of Hormones in Harmony Consulting (www.hormonesinharmony.com). She received her doctor of pharmacy degree from the University of California, San Francisco and is a board-certified pharmacist in California and Nevada and a member of the American Academy of Anti-Aging Medicine and the Institute for Integrative Medicine. She is also a former talk radio personality on KSRO 1350 AM in Santa Rosa, CA.

Amy has completed extensive training and continuing education in compounding pharmaceuticals and specializes in bioidentical hormone replacement therapy, functional medicine, derma- tology, and nutrition. Her consultations and seminar series are aimed at promoting longevity for both women and men. Her hormone consulting practice has evolved from meeting one-on-one with patients to teaching health care providers how to develop their own clinical hormone replacement and functional medicine programs. She also leads community group seminars for those seeking to learn the unbiased truth about bioidentical hormone replacement therapy and functional medicine.

Index

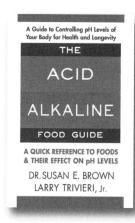

THE ACID-ALKALINE FOOD GUIDE

A Quick Reference to Foods & Their Effect on pH Levels

Dr. Susan E. Brown and Larry Trivieri, Jr.

The importance of acid-alkaline balance to good health is no secret. Thousands of people are trying to balance their body's pH level, but have had to rely on guides containing only a small number of foods. *The Acid-Alkaline Food Guide* is a complete resource for people who want to widen their food choices. After explaining how the acid-alkaline environment of the body is influenced by foods, this book lists thousands of foods—single foods, combination foods, and even fast foods—and their acid-alkaline effects.

$7.95 US • 208 pages • 4 x 7-inch mass paperback • ISBN 978-0-7570-0280-9

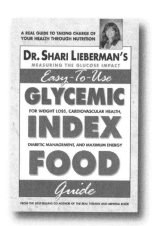

GLYCEMIC INDEX FOOD GUIDE

For Weight Loss, Cardiovascular Health, Diabetic Management, and Maximum Energy

Dr. Shari Lieberman

By indicating how quickly a given food triggers a rise in blood sugar, the glycemic index (GI) enables you to choose foods that can help you manage a variety of conditions and improve your overall health. Designed as an easy-to-use guide to the glycemic index, this book first answers commonly asked questions, ensuring that you truly understand the GI and know how to use it. It then provides both the glycemic index and the glycemic load for hundreds of foods and beverages.

$7.95 US • 160 pages • 4 x 7-inch mass paperback • ISBN 978-0-7570-0245-8

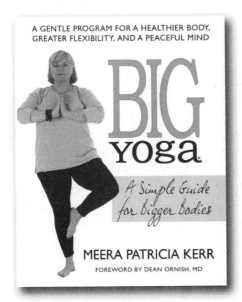

A GENTLE PROGRAM FOR A HEALTHIER BODY, GREATER FLEXIBILITY, AND A PEACEFUL MIND

MEERA PATRICIA KERR

FOREWORD BY DEAN ORNISH, MD

BIG YOGA
A Simple Guide for Bigger Bodies

Meera Patricia Kerr

Think yoga is only for skinny young things? Think again. To expert Meera Patricia Kerr, yoga can and should be used by everyone—*especially* plus-size individuals. In *Big Yoga*, Meera shares the unique yoga program she developed for all those who think that yoga is not for them.

Part One of *Big Yoga* begins with a clear explanation of what yoga is, what benefits it offers, and how it can fit into anyone's life. Included is an important discussion of self-image. The book goes on to provide practical information regarding clothing, mats, and suitable environments, and to emphasize the need to begin with care. Part Two offers over forty different exercises specifically designed to work with bigger bodies. In each case, the author explains the technique, details its advantages, and offers step-by-step instructions along with easy-to-follow photographs.

If you have thought that yoga is not for you, pick up *Big Yoga* and let Meera Kerr help you become more confident and relaxed than you may have ever thought possible.

$17.95 US • 240 pages • 7.5 x 9-inch quality paperback • ISBN 978-0-7570-0215-1

EMBRACING MENOPAUSE NATURALLY

Stories, Portraits, and Recipes

Gabriele Kushi

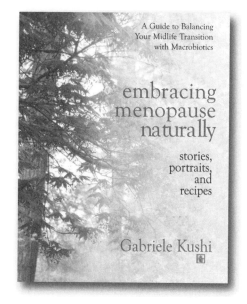

We are all too familiar with its symptoms: hot flashes, night sweats, and more. While menopause triggers many physical changes, it also brings forth spiritual issues that, for many women, mark a redefinition of the feminine self. To address the total impact of menopause, Gabriele Kushi has created a practical guide to dealing with this special time.

The author first provides a clear understanding of the overall process of menopause, from biological changes to emotional challenges. She then offers research-based nutritional guidelines that can help relieve menopausal symptoms, as well as healthful kitchen-tested recipes based on a natural foods diet. However, it is the stories and portraits of twenty menopausal women that are the heart and soul of the book. Here is a true companion for any woman who wants to nurture her own spiritual growth, adopt a natural foods diet, and enjoy good health throughout the midlife years.

$14.95 US • 160 pages • 7.5 x 9-inch quality paperback • ISBN 978-0-7570-0296-0

WHAT YOU MUST KNOW ABOUT WOMEN'S HORMONES

Your Guide to Natural Hormone Treatments for PMS, Menopause, Osteoporosis, PCOS, and More

Pamela Wartian Smith, MD, MPH

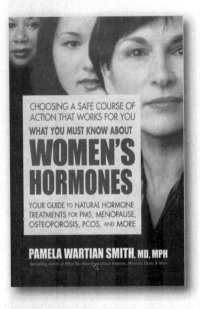

Hormonal imbalances can occur at any age—before, during, or after menopause—and for a variety of reasons. While most hormone-related problems are associated with menopause, fluctuating hormonal levels can also cause a variety of other conditions, and for some women, the effects can be truly debilitating. *What You Must Know About Women's Hormones* is a clear guide to the treatment of hormonal irregularities without the health risks associated with standard hormone replacement therapy.

Part I describes the body's own hormones, looking at their functions and the problems that can occur if they are not at optimal levels. Part II focuses on the most common problems that arise from hormonal imbalances, such as PMS, hot flashes, and endometriosis. Lastly, Part III details hormone replacement therapy, focusing on the difference between natural and synthetic hormone treatments.

Whether you are looking for help with menopausal symptoms or you simply want to enjoy vibrant health, *What You Must Know About Women's Hormones* can make a profound difference in your life.

$17.95 US • 256 pages • 6 x 9-inch quality paperback • ISBN 978-0-7570-0307-3

For more information about our books, visit our website at www.squareonepublishers.com